MONOGRAPHS OF THE PHYSIOLOGICAL SOCIETY

Editors: H. Dawson, A. D. M. Greenfield,
R. Whittam, D. G. Brindley

Number 20 MECHANISMS OF URINE CONCENTRATION
AND DILUTION IN MAMMALS

MONOGRAPHS OF THE PHYSIOLOGICAL SOCIETY

Volumes marked ★ are now out of print.

MECHANISMS OF URINE CONCENTRATION AND DILUTION IN MAMMALS

by

S. E. DICKER

M.D., Ph.D., D.Sc.

*Professor of Physiology, Chelsea College
and Honorary Research Assistant, University College
University of London*

LONDON
EDWARD ARNOLD (PUBLISHERS) LTD

Printed in Great Britain by
The Camelot Press Ltd., London and Southampton

To

M. G. E.

F. R. W.

H. H.

in all friendship

'We ought not to reject the ancient art as non-existent, or on the ground that its method of inquiry is faulty, just because it has not attained exactness in every detail, but much rather because it has been able by reasoning to rise from deep ignorance to approximately perfect accuracy, I think we ought to admire the discoveries as the work, not of chance, but of inquiry rightly and correctly conducted.'—*Hippocrates* (460–355 B.C.)*

* *Translated by Jones, W. H. S. (1923).*

PREFACE

THE study of the mechanism of urine concentration and dilution has advanced greatly in the last decades due to an increasing awareness of the wealth of information which can be derived from it. The concepts introduced by Homer Smith, supported by the results from early micropuncture techniques and the appraisal of comparative physiology, were the basis of the study. It is hoped that the present book will serve both as an introduction for research workers interested in the subject and as a help for those who, though already familiar with it, wish to be informed of more recent developments.

The title of the book sets no apparent limits to its scope. While in the process of writing it, I became aware that I would be able to deal with only some aspects of the problem. The decision to deal with some and to omit other views was my own. The justification for doing so can be found in prefaces to previous monographs in this series, where it was pointed out that monographs are not reviews. Whereas in the latter no personal opinion is expected, in the former the reader looks for the opinion of one worker in a specialized field. This involved choice. Choice, however, has to be justified since the author must be aware that 'his monograph will be read and critized by experts, to whom he must supply sufficient reason for adopting one interpretation and excluding others' (O'Connor, 1962). Whether I have succeeded in this only the reader will decide.

While I must alone bear the responsibility for its shortcomings, it is only right to state that this book would never have been written at all had I not been introduced to the study of renal physiology while still an undergraduate student. This goes back to the time when I was allowed to work with the late Professor J. Demoor in Brussels. But the real assistance and encouragement in the study of renal physiology I owe to three friends who have never failed me and have inspired and guided me throughout the best part of my life. To these I would like to express my very special gratitude: F. R. Winton, Professor Emeritus of London University, M. Grace Eggleton, former Reader in Physiology at University College London, and H. Heller, Professor of Pharmacology at the University of Bristol.

There are many other friends, too numerous to be mentioned by name, to whom I owe much: technicians, students and research workers, some of whom now occupy positions of eminence in their own field of investigation. They have all, whether they knew it or not, helped in their own capacity and collaborated in the development of my work and made it possible for me to write this Monograph. None of them, however, do I wish to burden with responsibility for any views advanced in this book, except where expressly stated.

I want to single out, in my expression of indebtedness, Dr. M. Grace Eggleton, who has not only made suggestions for improving obscure passages, but offered to prepare the Index and correct the proof.

I should like to thank Professor Annie B. Elliott, Dr. Venetia King and Dr. D. Rosen for reading the whole or part of the manuscript and making helpful suggestions and criticisms.

My gratitude goes also to my wife who has assisted me with the preparation of the book and who had to live with the manuscript for so long.

This book would never have been written without the inexhaustible patience and energy of my secretary, Mrs. P. Diboll. I am indebted to Mr. J. Thynne and Mrs. B. Thompson for their help in the preparation of figures.

I should like to thank Mr. C. F. A. Marmoy, librarian of the Thane Library at University College London, for his help in tracing references.

Acknowledgement for permission to reproduce published figures is due also to the editors and publishers of the following journals and books:

The American Journal of Physiology (American Physiological Society), *The Journal of Comparative Biochemistry and Physiology* (Pergamon Press), *Science* (Washington, D.C.), *Pflügers Archiv für die gesamte Physiologie des Menschen und der Tiere* (Springer-

Verlag), *Helvetica Physiologia et Pharmacolia* (Schwabe & Co.) data from J. Schnarman's paper at the 6th Symposium of the Society of Nephrology (Vienna 1968), *The Journal of Physiology* (Cambridge), *The Journal of Cell Biology* (Rockefeller University Press, New York), *Endocrinologia Experimentalis* (U.S.S.R.) and E. & S. Livingstone Ltd. for a figure from Bell, Davidson and Scarborough's *Textbook of Physiology and Biochemistry*.

Finally, I am most grateful to Mr. R. E. Strange of Arnolds for his help and collaboration in the setting of the text.

CONTENTS

I

'CHAPTER ONE'

THE separation of a glomerular ultrafiltrate from the plasma forms a convenient starting point for discussion of how the kidneys regulate the water balance of the body. The ultrafiltrate is essentially a protein-free fluid iso-osmotic with the plasma, as shown by Wearn & Richards (1924) who used Chambers' micro-dissection technique for the collection of fluid from Bowman's capsule to determine the composition of the capsular fluid of the frog (*Rana pipiens*), the mud-puppy (*Necturus maculosus*) and other amphibians. They found that the glomerular fluid normally contains no protein, but contains glucose and chloride though the urine in the bladder is free of glucose and poor in chloride. Subsequent investigators showed that in both the frog and *Necturus* the osmotic pressure of the capsular fluid and the blood plasma from which it is formed are the same, as is also the electrical conductivity (Bayliss & Walker, 1930; Walker, 1930). The chloride content of the glomerular ultrafiltrate in both animals was found to be a little higher than in plasma, as would be expected from the Donnan equilibrium (Wearn & Richards, 1925; Freeman, Livingston & Richards, 1930; Richards, 1934; Westfall, Findley & Richards, 1934; Richards & Walker, 1936). Urea, glucose, in-organic phosphate, creatinine and uric acid were found in the capsular fluid of the frog and of the snake in the same concentra-tion as in plasma (Walker & Elsom, 1930; Walker & Reisinger, 1933; Walker, 1933; Bordley & Richards, 1933; Bordley, Hendrix & Richards, 1933) and finally the ultrafiltrate was shown to have the same pH as the plasma (Montgomery, 1935; Pierce & Montgomery, 1935).

Direct analysis of glomerular filtrate in mammals was achieved later, but indirect evidence, drawn from observations of the effect of perfusion and of ureter pressure on urine formation, had already

I

led to similar conclusions. The first experiments along this line were performed by Starling in 1899. This was followed by a series of publications, among which those of Henderson (1905), Bainbridge & Evans (1914), Starling & Verney (1925), Winton (1931*a*, *b*, *c*) and Bayliss, Kerridge & Russell (1933) should be mentioned. They all supported the hypothesis of glomerular filtration. Subsequently, Walker, Bott, Oliver & McDowell (1941) extended the micropuncture technique initiated by Richards and his collaborators as early as 1923 (Richards, 1929) to the rat, guinea pig and opossum. Although glomerular puncture is more difficult in mammals than in amphibians because most of the glomeruli are located below the surface of the cortex, it could be shown that the capsular fluid in these rodents had the same characteristics as in amphibians. It is essentially protein free, it has the same osmotic pressure as the blood plasma, and contains glucose creatinine, sodium, chloride and phosphate in the amounts expected in a fluid formed by ultrafiltration (Walker & Oliver, 1941).

In man, urine flow normally varies between about 20 ml./min and

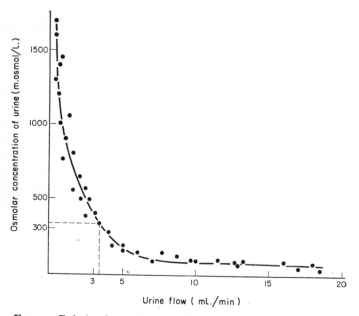

FIG. 1.1 Relation between concentration of urine and urine flow in man.

TABLE 1.1

Values of C_{osm} in human subjects

Subject I			Subject II			Subject III			Subject IV		
V (ml./min)	U_{osm}/P_{osm}	C_{osm} (ml./min)	V (ml./min)	U_{osm}/P_{osm}	C_{osm} (ml./min)	V (ml./min)	U_{osm}/P_{osm}	C_{osm} (ml./min)	V (ml./min)	U_{osm}/P_{osm}	C_{osm} (ml./min)
0·33	5·14	1·70	0·60	4·20	2·52	2·40	1·52	3·65	1·20	2·90	3·48
0·73	4·39	3·20	0·93	2·26	2·10	3·10	1·05	3·26	1·60	1·64	2·62
2·00	1·96	3·92	2·40	1·19	2·86	5·07	0·47	2·38	7·67	0·44	3·37
3·30	1·00	3·30	3·10	0·96	2·98	11·46	0·27	3·09	12·87	0·22	2·83
5·00	0·57	2·85	4·00	0·77	3·08	12·67	0·24	3·04	15·93	0·17	2·70
9·90	0·38	3·27	4·26	0·59	2·51	13·33	0·23	3·06	17·50	0·16	2·80
10·00	0·33	3·80	4·90	0·53	2·60	—	—	—	—	—	—

Mean ±S.E. (26) = 2·86±0·163 ml./min

The data were obtained from a class experiment. The subjects were 4 healthy students who drank amounts of water varying between 500 to 1500 ml. water. Urine was collected at ten-minute intervals throughout the experiment.

0·3 ml./min. The osmolar concentration of urine excreted at low rates is much higher than that of the plasma or the glomerular filtrate; likewise, at high rates of flow, urine is much more dilute than the original ultrafiltrate (Fig 1.1). By expressing the osmotic pressure of urine in terms of the concentration of osmotically active constituents, it may vary from about 30, or less at a flow of 17 ml., to about 1300–1500 m-osmole/l. at a flow of 0·5 ml./min. Between these extremes there will be a rate at which urine has the same osmotic pressure as that of the glomerular filtrate. In the example represented in Table 1.1, this is about 3·0 ml./min. In terms of work, when urine is iso-osmotic with plasma the osmotic work of the kidney is nil. The osmotically active constituents of the urine will then require the simultaneous excretion of a volume of water sufficient to contain them in a solution of the same osmotic pressure as that of plasma. Since this volume, expressed in ml./min represents the rate at which osmotically active substances are cleared from the plasma, it has been called the 'osmolar clearance', or C_{osm}.

Values of osmolar clearance are calculated in the same way as any other clearance; thus:

$$C_{osm} = \frac{U_{osm}}{P_{osm}} \times V \qquad (1.1)$$

where U_{osm} is the concentration of urine (m-osmole/l.) and P_{osm} that of plasma (m-osmole/l.), both values being derived from the depression of the freezing point of either urine or plasma, and V is the urine flow (ml./min).

Values for osmolar clearances are not affected by changes of urine flow (Table 1.1); they may, however, vary with changes in filtration rate. According to Smith (1956) the basal osmolar clearance in man ranges from 1 to 3% of the glomerular filtration rate, depending on the quantities of urea, NaCl, $NaHCO_3$ and other substances excreted.

It is of interest to see what happens during a fully developed 'osmotic diuresis'. This is a diuresis produced as the result of an osmotic effect. It does not involve the kidneys in additional osmotic work. It occurs whenever solutes in the tubules are concentrated enough to exert an osmotic effect. A typical example of this is the diuresis following intravenous infusion of mannitol.

Mannitol is filtered by the glomeruli, but passes along the renal tubules without undergoing appreciable reabsorption. As the load in the tubules increases, the proportion of filtered water normally reabsorbed will fall; in other words, as the rate of total solute excretion increases, its concentration in the urine decreases until finally it approximates to that of the plasma (Bull, 1956). In these circumstances and owing entirely to an osmotic effect the U_{osm}/P_{osm} ratio will be nearing unity and the value of osmolar clearance will be equal to that of urine flow. It follows that whenever the urine flow is equal to the osmolar clearance, the net renal operation consists merely in the excretion of a fraction of osmotically unchanged glomerular filtrate. In normal circumstances, urine flow rarely exceeds 10% of the glomerular filtrate, but during 'osmotic diuresis' it can be greater. For instance, following the intravenous injection of sodium sulphate in dogs, a urine flow equivalent to about 60% of the glomerular filtration rate has been observed (Shannon, 1938); and Smith (1943) after prolonged glucose infusion in man reported a urine flow approaching 40% of the filtration rate. Though in the normal course of events, the rate of urine flow is different from that of osmolar clearance, this is even more marked in two extreme cases when the subject is either hydropoenic or overhydrated (West, Kaplan, Fomon & Rapoport, 1952).

When a subject is hydrated the urine flow increases markedly. This usually occurs without significant changes in the glomerular filtration rate or in osmolar clearance. As the osmolar clearance represents the rate at which osmotically active substances are cleared from the plasma simultaneously with a volume of water sufficient to contain them in a solution iso-osmotic with the plasma, any surplus of water which will account for a diuresis can be considered as solute-free distilled water. In other words, during a water diuresis, the urine may be considered as being formed by a mixture of osmotically 'obligated' water, equal in amount to the osmolar clearance, and of solute-free water (Wesson & Anslow, 1948, 1952; Smith, 1956). Since the urine flow (ml./min) excreted during a water diuresis is equal to the sum of the osmolar clearance C_{osm} (ml./min) and the excess of free water (ml./min) or C_{H2O}, this can be expressed as:

$$V = C_{osm} + C_{H2O} \qquad (1.2)$$

and the amount of solute-free water expressed in terms of clearance will be:

$$C_{H_2O} = V - C_{osm} \qquad (1.3)$$

or

$$C_{H_2O} = \left(1 - \frac{U_{osm}}{P_{osm}}\right) \times V \qquad (1.4)$$

where $V =$ urine flow (ml./min); U_{osm} and P_{osm} are the concentrations of solutes as expressed by the depression of freezing point of urine and plasma; C_{osm} is the osmolar clearance (ml./min) and C_{H_2O} the free water clearance (ml./min).

Thus the clearance of free water is derived from the estimation of another clearance, the osmolar clearance, and cannot be estimated from the U/P ratio alone because there is no osmotically free water in the plasma. As Smith (1956) remarked: 'The kidneys excrete it only by generating it (as in the case of ammonia) and in this respect, the term clearance in describing the rate of excretion of free water departs somewhat from its conventional meaning.'

Values of C_{H_2O} will be positive whenever the osmotic pressure of the urine is lower than that of the plasma or of the glomerular filtrate, as during a water diuresis. In theory, a positive free-water clearance could be brought about in two ways: by a tubular secretion of water, which would be added effectively to the iso-osmotic glomerular filtrate, or by a tubular reabsorption of osmotically active solutes without their equivalent of water. The first hypothesis would require that somewhere along the renal tubules water should be secreted actively; the other, that solutes such as Na^+ and Cl^- should be transported actively through membranes virtually impermeable to water.

An interesting question is whether the free-water clearance can be increased by administration of diuretic substances. Generally speaking, all diuretics exert directly or indirectly an osmotic effect which results either from an increased load of solutes which has to be excreted, such as during intravenous infusions of mannitol or urea, or from the inhibition of reabsorption of ions such as sodium or chloride. During diuresis following the drinking of a large volume of water (1·5 to 2·0 l.) in man, the free-water clearance increases steadily with the urine flow and may reach nearly 12% of the glomerular filtration rate (Smith, 1947). This can also be shown on a non-anaesthetized dog. The amount

of water per unit body weight tolerated by a dog is 3–4 times
that of man. Under laboratory conditions a dog can be given
75 ml. water/kg body weight by stomach tube. In one such experiment, the urine flow averaged 9·4 ml./min and the calculated
free-water clearance amounted to 8·0 ml./min. When during the
water diuresis the dog was given an intravenous infusion of
2·0 g urea/kg, the urine flow increased from an average of 9·4 ml.
to 17·9 ml./min, but the value of the free-water clearance remained
very much the same as during the control period. If the urea was
replaced by a mercurial diuretic, there was likewise an increase of
urine flow above that of a water diuresis. Values for free-water
clearance either remained substantially unaltered or they decreased
slightly. Similar findings were observed when furosemide or
ethacrynic acid were given to man during a water diuresis
(Puschett & Goldberg, 1968) or when hydrochlorothiazide was
administered orally to fully hydrated rats or fowl (Dicker & Eggleton, 1964b; Dicker, Eggleton & Haslam, 1966). Everything then
suggests that there may be an upper limit to the amount of free water
that can be excreted. Since, however, there is no clear evidence
that this amount of water is added to the iso-osmotic urine in
the distal convoluted tube, it must be assumed that it is produced
by a definite quantity of osmotically active solutes being reabsorbed.

    So far, the discussion has evolved in terms of changes of osmotic
pressures which may occur in the urine during its passage from the
glomeruli to the ureter. The way in which these changes are
brought about must now be examined. As fluid leaves the glomeruli
and enters the proximal tubules, it undergoes a series of important
changes. Glucose is withdrawn (Walker & Hudson, 1937a;
Walker et al., 1941; Malvin, Wilde & Sullivan, 1958), amino acids
are reabsorbed (Eaton, Ferguson & Beyer, 1946; Ferguson,
Eaton & Ashman, 1947; Pitts, Brown & Samiy, 1959) and so is
most of the sodium chloride content. From micropuncture studies
in rat and guinea-pig, it would appear that some 80% of the
glomerular filtrate is reabsorbed, though the urine in this part of
the nephron remains iso-osmotic with the plasma. The absence of
changes of the osmotic pressure of the fluid in the proximal tubule
in spite of its reduction in volume could be attributed either to the
primary movement of water followed by NaCl, or alternatively to
the movement of NaCl followed by water.

    Wesson & Anslow (1948, 1952) and Wesson, Anslow & Smith

(1948) induced an osmotic diuresis in dogs by intravenous infusion of hypertonic solutions of mannitol. The resultant urine flow was approximately two thirds of the rate of glomerular filtration. It was assumed that such high flows of urine precluded any significant alteration of the urine by the distal part of the nephrons, and therefore its composition was accepted as similar to that of the fluid as it leaves the proximal convoluted tubes. The interesting point was that though the total osmotic pressure of the urine was very similar to that of the plasma the composition of the urine was different: it contained 65% of the filtered water but no more than about 25% of the filtered sodium. The fact that proportionally so much less sodium than water reached the bladder was taken as evidence that the reabsorption of this ion in the proximal tubule was independent of that of water.

Smith and his collaborators never investigated the real role of the loops of Henle; in their view the thin limb of the loop acts as a site for osmotic equilibration, allowing if necessary diffusion of water to occur so as to rectify any deviation from iso-osmoticity. Thus, in Homer Smith's view, the process of glomerular filtration, of proximal reabsorption, of equilibration in the loop of Henle, all resulted in the formation of an iso-osmotic fluid reaching the distal tubule; and it was to the collecting ducts that were attributed the rather complicated mechanisms which determine ultimately the concentration, dilution and composition of the urine.

According to Brodsky & Rapoport (1951) and to Brodsky, Austing, Moxley & Grubbs (1953) dilution of the urine is achieved by secretion of water to the fluid in the distal tubules. Since, however, during a water diuresis, the urine is virtually sodium free, it could be argued that dilution was achieved by the removal of osmotically active solutes. According to the latter hypothesis, the epithelium of the distal tubule would be impermeable to water so as to prevent any water from following in the wake of actively transported sodium.

If tubular fluid is diluted by active reabsorption of solute, without accompanying water, the elaboration of a hypertonic urine involves removal of water without solute, and the free-water clearance becomes negative. Rather than speaking of a negative clearance, the deficit of water $T_{H_2O}^c$ can be expressed as

$$T_{H_2O}^c \ (\text{ml./min}) = C_{osm} \ (\text{ml./min}) - V \ (\text{ml./min}) \qquad (1.5)$$

When sufficient antidiuretic hormone is administered to man during a water diuresis, so as to reduce his urine flow and concentrate his urine, there is no significant change in the output of sodium. Hence the rate of sodium reabsorption along the whole length of the nephron remains unchanged. Since the rate of reabsorption of sodium affects the dilution of urine, and since this seems to be unaffected during antidiuresis, the question arises as to what is the functional and physiological relation between the process of dilution and that of concentration? In other words, does the reabsorption of water without solute take place through the same tubular epithelium which in the absence of the antidiuretic hormone is almost completely impermeable to water? Smith considered this to be improbable and preferred to locate the diluting mechanism in the distal tubule whereas that for concentrating would be in the collecting ducts. Smith found support for his views in clinical observations which showed that during the evolution of chronic renal disease, the loss of ability to concentrate urine precedes the loss of capacity for water diuresis, and that during the recovery phase of acute renal insufficiency, the power to concentrate urine is the last to return (Smith, 1952). His views received further support when micropuncture techniques revealed the composition of tubular fluid in the different parts of the nephron. Walker et al. in 1941 had noted that fluid in the early part of the distal convoluted tubule of the rat was invariably *hypotonic* to plasma, an observation which was ignored until rediscovered fifteen years later by Wirz (1956). During water diuresis, the hypotonicity of the fluid in the distal tubule is maintained or even slightly increased along the whole course of the distal tubule. During antidiuresis, however, the fluid becomes more concentrated as it proceeds along the length of the distal portion of the tubule, but *never* exceeds iso-osmoticity with plasma or glomerular filtrate. Since the urine in the ureters can be considerably more concentrated than the plasma, the ultimate process of concentration must be located in the collecting ducts. Wirz's observations in 1956, supported by those of Gottschalk & Mylle (1959), unexpectedly afforded a solid experimental support for Smith's hypothesis that concentration and dilution are functions located at different sites within the nephron.

There is an interesting corollary to this concept of functional independence. According to Smith, the removal of solute-free water is a continuous autonomous process, uncontrolled by the antidiuretic hormone, and therefore existing even in its absence (Smith, 1951, 1952, 1956). Already in 1942 Shannon had observed that dogs with experimentally induced diabetes insipidus, with a low glomerular filtration rate and suffering from dehydration, were able to produce hypertonic urine. At first, this was attributed to the possible release of small amounts of antidiuretic hormone since complete surgical hypophysectomy is seldom achieved. de Wardener & Del Greco (1955), Del Greco & de Wardener (1956) and Berliner & Davidson (1957), working independently, showed, however, that urine more concentrated than plasma can be excreted without any evidence of release of the antidiuretic hormone. Dogs undergoing water diuresis were prepared so as to enable separate urine collection from each kidney. When a steady flow of dilute urine was established, a clamp was applied to one renal artery. This resulted in a unilateral reduction of glomerular filtration rate, accompanied by a unilateral reduction of urine flow (Leaf, Kerr, Wrong & Chatillon, 1954; Sellwood & Verney, 1955), but the urine excreted from the kidney with a reduced filtration rate was hypertonic to plasma. The rate of urine excretion from the unclamped kidney remained unaffected and so was its dilution (Berliner & Davidson, 1957). Similar observations were made in water-loaded rats under ethanol anaesthesia which were in a state resembling that of diabetes insipidus (Dicker, 1957). Though the excretion of hypertonic urine in the absence of antidiuretic hormone supports the idea of Smith of an autonomous process of water reabsorption, it must be pointed out that in these experiments urinary concentrations in excess of 600 m-osmole/l. were not obtained, though in normal circumstances, a dog can excrete urine with concentration of the order of 2000 m-osmole/l.

Since the kidney alone can elaborate a urine more concentrated than plasma, how can the antidiuretic hormone increase its ability to do so? According to Smith and his co-workers, the process of water reabsorption in the proximal and distal tubules is similar in so far as that in both the movement of water follows passively that of sodium. There is a difference, however: whereas in the proximal tubule the movements of sodium and water occur through an epithelium permeable to water, and are independent of the presence or absence of the antidiuretic hormone; in the distal tubule, sodium transport is through an epithelium normally impermeable to water and is accompanied by an iso-osmotic movement of water only when the antidiuretic hormone is present. Thus, according to this hypothesis, the production of hypertonic urine proceeds in two phases: during the first, there is a passive diffusion of osmotically free water made available by the active reabsorption of sodium; during the second, there is a further reabsorption of water from the residual isotonic fluid, rendering the tubular content hypertonic to plasma. Both phases would be possible as a result of a change of permeability of the epithelium to water produced by the antidiuretic hormone.

In the second phase, during which the process of concentration occurs, water must be transported from an area of higher concentration to an area of isotonicity. This as visualized by Smith (1947) and by Wesson & Anslow (1948) is an active process. Since it is supposed to be an active process, it should be subject to limits like any other active transport. Experimental evidence on man and animals supports this view. The highest urinary concentration that man can achieve is of the order of 1400 m-osmole/l., during which the U_{osm}/P_{osm} ratio is 4 to 5. In other words, there would appear to be a limiting gradient against which water can be transported only in such amounts as to render the urine 4 to 5 times as concentrated as plasma. In animals, these figures may be higher: the highest osmolarity of the urine of the dog is 5–6 times, of the rat 7–9 times and of the desert rat 16–20 times that of the blood plasma.

The fact that there appears to be in each species a limit to the amount by which the urine can be concentrated would be in agreement with the existence of a limiting mechanism to water transport. Similar conclusions were reached from experiments on dogs (Page & Reem, 1952), on seals (Page, Scott-Baker, Zak, Becker & Baxter, 1954), and on rats (Dicker, 1957). Besides the limit of a maximal gradient, there would appear to be a limit to the amount of water that can be transported to produce a concentrated urine. Zak, Brun & Smith (1954) infused hydropoenic human subjects for several hours with an hypertonic solution of mannitol together with vasopressin. They observed an osmotic diuresis with maximum urine flows of the order 32–35 ml./min. Though the glomerular filtration rate, as estimated from inulin clearance, remained practically unchanged, the osmolar clearance values increased steadily and were consistently higher than the calculated values for an iso-osmotic state by an amount of about 5·2 ml./min. Thus, an infusion of a hypertonic solution of mannitol produced a maximum concentration of urine either by the re-absorption of a fixed amount of water from or by addition of a constant amount of osmotically active solutes to the iso-osmotic tubular fluid. Since in these experiments the main constituents accounting for the osmotic pressure of the urine were mannitol and sodium, and since neither mannitol nor sodium is secreted into the tubular urine, the concentration of urine could be achieved only by transport of water. The amount of water transported was the same irrespective of the urine flow. As a matter of fact, for any urine flow in excess of 5 ml./min the amount of water transported, T_{H_2O}, was not only found to be constant but maximum ($T^c_{mH_2O}$). Thus, the concentrating mechanism would appear to consist of a constant reabsorptive process which removes water at an approximately fixed rate ($T^c_{H_2O}$) from the iso-osmotic tubular fluid, this proceeding as long as the volume of the latter exceeds the value for $T^c_{mH_2O}$. This interpretation affords an explanation of what happens during osmotic diuresis, whether the antidiuretic hormone is present or not. The loading of the kidneys with a solute such as mannitol, which is not reabsorbed by the tubules, produces a decrease of the amount of sodium reabsorbed by either the proximal or the distal convoluted tubules. If less sodium is re-absorbed, there will be a smaller amount of free water. Since the action of the antidiuretic hormone is to produce iso-osmotic reabsorption of free water, it is clear that no amount of the anti-diuretic hormone will be able to effect the concentration of the fluid in the distal tubule above isotonicity. As the rate of solute excretion increases, the ultimate concentration of the urine will approach isotonicity in an asymptotic fashion. This can be readily visualized by reference to equations (1) to (4) as, by substituting $T^c_{mH_2O}$ for $T^c_{H_2O}$, we shall have

$$\frac{U_{osm}}{P_{osm}} = \left(1 + \frac{T^c_{mH_2O}}{V}\right) \tag{1.6}$$

As $T^c_{mH_2O}$ is constant by definition and V increases progressively, the fraction $T^c_{mH_2O}/V$ must become correspondingly smaller until the U_{osm}/P_{osm} approaches 1 asymptotically.

This is in brief what can now be considered the 'classical'

concept of the mechanism of urine concentration and dilution. It rests on the postulate that water is actively transported against an osmotic gradient and that the renal medulla is essentially iso-osmotic with plasma.

It has been claimed that active transport of water is the source of the hypotonic urine in aglomerular fishes (Edwards & Condorelli, 1928; Marshall, 1930), and that it takes place against an osmotic gradient in the small intestine of the rat (Fisher, 1955; Parsons & Wingate, 1961). Its existence and the ways in which it might operate have been investigated and discussed by several authors. Suppose that the sequence of oxidative processes which occur at one end of a secreting cell cease and that a substance X of low molecular weight is formed, but is unable to penetrate the cell membrane. This will result in a certain amount of water being drawn into the cell from the outside. If now this substance became completely oxidized to carbon dioxide and water, the water drawn in at one end would pass out at the other end. Thus water would pass from a solution of greater solute concentration to one of less, contrary to its own activity gradient. It has been calculated that if such a process obtained in the distal tubules of the mammalian kidney, each millilitre of water traversing the cell would be accompanied by 1·5 milliosmoles of solute which would have to be fully oxidized. This would involve a stoicheiometric relation between the rate of oxygen consumption and that of water transport, and as Bayliss (1959) remarked: 'Even with the most favourable assumptions, it is calculated that the active absorption of water alone would use as much oxygen in a given time as is observed to be used by the whole of both kidneys, leaving none for the many other kinds of secretion.'

This difficulty, however, would be avoided in the 'osmotic diffusion pump' (Frank & Mayer, 1947). In this model, the osmotically active solute formed at one end of the cell loses its osmotic activity at the other end by being either synthesized or polymerized into much larger molecules, which then diffuse back to the entry side, where they are split into their original components. The splitting of the polymer will entail reactions which in turn will involve the reduction of molecular oxygen. Though in this model there is no need for a stoicheiometric relation between the amount of oxygen reduced and that of the 'carrier' substance polymerized or split, there is an energetic limiting value to the system. There is, however, another objection. In the 'osmotic diffusion pump', the carrier, whether polymerized or metabolized, is supposed to diffuse across the cell, carrying with it the water molecules which are transported. To be efficient, the rate at which the carrier diffuses must be related to the rate of water transport and to the concentration difference against which the transport occurs. But whereas the rate of diffusion of the carrier will be determined by the difference in concentrations between the two ends of the cell and the length of the latter, the rate of water transport will be determined by the effective concentration difference across the semi-permeable membrane and its permeability to water (Bayliss, 1959). Even if there were a relation between the rate of diffusion of the carrier and that of water transport, the metabolic processes involved make the hypothesis untenable. It has been calculated that for the metabolic processes to proceed at a rate sufficient to maintain the steady state of concentration difference across the cell, the metabolic rate of each cell involved in this mechanism would be some 1000 times greater than that of any known living cell (Brodsky, Rehm, Dennis & Miller, 1955). Thus such a pump could work only if the rate of diffusion of the carrier substance could be reduced 1000-fold or so.

Water can be transported during electro-osmosis. Electro-osmosis involves not merely the presence of a potential difference, but the passage of an electric current. So long as there is a flux of ions, active or passive, there will also be a flow of current; electric charges carried by water molecules will then contribute to this current in the same way as the ions. It has been suggested that the electro-osmotic transport of water will not occur through the same parts of the membrane as does the transport of ions, or that it may occur through the cement substance which lies between cells. According to Höber (1947) the conditions for electro-osmosis would be analogous if not similar to those leading to 'anomalous osmosis'. In the systems in which anomalous osmosis has been studied a steady state may be maintained by some form of active return of the diffusing electrolyte into the more concentrated solution from which it comes (Bayliss, 1959). It is, however, doubtful whether electro-osmotic effects can play a role in the transport of water in the kidney.

Though the concept of urine concentration, as expounded by Homer Smith and his associates, could have withstood minor criticisms (Lamdin, 1959), it was unable to resist the evidence that iso-osmoticity did not exist in the renal medulla. Faced with this new evidence, Smith refused to commit himself and remained to the last deliberately vague about the specific mechanism of urine concentration. His theory, besides being 'enticing as a speculation' (Smith, 1951), and in spite of minor modifications, remained based on the assumption that during the elaboration of hypertonic urine, all the constituents of the medulla with the exception of the collecting ducts were iso-osmotic with plasma—hypertonicity of the urine being brought about by a transfer of pure water from the ducts into the iso-osmotic medulla (Smith, 1947). Presumably the vasa recta, having taken up this water, were carrying it off for ultimate redistribution within the total body water. Assuming that the rate and volume of blood flow were large enough, it might be conceivable that interstitial and intracapillary osmotic pressure would not be measurably lowered and that isotonicity might be maintained.

It may be appropriate to quote from Homer Smith (1951). Talking of the history of renal physiology he wrote, 'It has been a history of rival theories, each based on inconclusive evidence. Its errors have been compounded by oversimplification in the matter of theory and underexamination in the matter of critical investigation. Renal physiology has now passed into a quantitative phase where unsupported speculation and empirical description are no longer warranted.'

2

RENAL STRUCTURE AND ABILITY TO CONCENTRATE URINE

DEVELOPMENTALLY the kidney is derived from the surface of the coelomic cavity and is thus a mesodermic organ. Each kidney is made up of a large number of units, called nephrons, all basically similar in structure and presumably also similar in function. The number of nephrons in each kidney has been counted. According to Cushny (1926) Peter (1909) thought that the dog's kidney had 300,000 units; whereas in the pig the number of nephrons were of the order of 500,000 and in man 4,500,000. In the adult rat, each kidney appears to have about 30,000 glomeruli (Kittelson, 1917; Arataki, 1926; Rytand, 1938). According to Smith (1951), however, the number of nephrons in one kidney in the rabbit is 207,000; in the dog 408,000; in the pig 1,193,000 and in man 1,095,000.

Each nephron consists of a renal or Malpighian corpuscle (glomerulus and capsule of Bowman) and a long unbranched tubule running a devious route through the cortex and medulla to end with many others in a collecting tube which opens into the pelvis of the kidney. The tubule has its origin in the capsule of Bowman. In most mammals, it 'doubles and twists (proximal convoluted tube) in the neighbourhood of the capsule, and then issues in a straight length directed towards the pelvis of the kidney. After running for some distance through the medulla, it doubles back (loop of Henle) to the neighbourhood of the capsule again in a straight course, and passing through a second though shorter series of convolutions (distal convoluted tubule) ends in the collecting tubule' (Cushny, 1926). In lower vertebrates there is little or no evidence of a loop of Henle. In the turtle's kidney, the nephron is shorter than in mammals, the loop of Henle being absent or very short. In the frog, there is no true kidney corresponding to the mammalian organ: the glomerulus is very small and there is no loop of Henle. The glomeruli of birds and reptiles consist of a capillary tuft with four short capillary loops only; as for the loop of Henle in birds, it is short and ill-developed (Marshall & Smith, 1930) and when present exists in some but not all nephrons (Smith, 1951).

The localization of the different segments of the nephrons in the kidney is the base for dividing the organ into cortex, medulla and papilla. The cortex contains all the glomeruli, the proximal and the distal convoluted tubules as well as the beginning of the collecting tubes. The medulla consists essentially of the loop of Henle, the limbs of which run more or less parallel towards the tip of the pyramids, together with the collecting tubes.

Views as to the actual limits of each portion of the tubules, especially the distal part, seem to vary. According to Smith (1937; 1951), the tubular portion of the nephron can be divided into three segments: (1) the proximal tubule which includes both the pars convoluta and the pars recta as far as the transition in the medulla to the thin segment of the loop of Henle, (2) the thin segment and (3) the distal tubule which includes the ascending limb of the loop as well as the pars convoluta. For Pitts (1963) and Clapp & Robinson (1966) the loop of Henle includes the pars recta of the proximal tubule, the thin segment and the pars recta of the distal tubule. As for the distal tubule, it starts at a site where the tubule, after it has doubled back, comes in contact with the glomerulus from which it originated (Peter, 1909; Hüber, 1917; Sperber, 1944; Pitts, 1963).

The loops of Henle are not all of the same length; some are short, others are long; in some animals the loop is reduced to a thin segment localized in the cortex, whilst in others it does not exist (Peter, 1909; Sperber, 1944; Maximow & Bloom, 1952). In some mammals like *Psammonys* all nephrons have long loops of Henle (Sperber, 1944); in others such as *Aplodontia*, the majority of nephrons have loops which do not reach the medulla (Pfeiffer, Nungesser, Iverson & Wallerius, 1960) (Fig. 2.1).

The medulla can be divided into the external medulla, itself sub-divided in superficial and inner layers, and the internal medulla. The external medulla contains the thick ascending limbs of the loops, while the thin segments of the loops are located in the internal medulla. The lower limit of the superficial layer of the

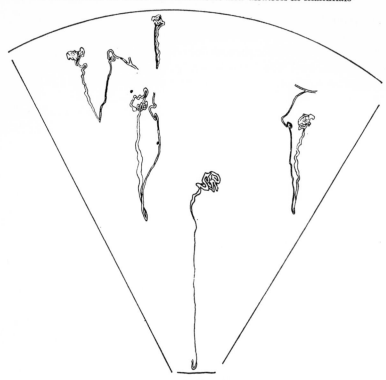

FIG. 2.1 Drawings of isolated nephrons dissected from the kidney of *Aplodontia rufa* after maceration in concentrated HCl. The nephrons are drawn in the relative position which they occupy in the kidney. Starting from the top there is a cortical nephron, a nephron with a short loop, two nephrons with a loop of intermediate length and one nephron only with a long loop. The cortical nephron has no thin segment; others have only short thin segments, with the loop occurring in a thick limb which becomes the ascending limb of the loop of Henle (after Nungesser & Pfeiffer, 1965).

medulla corresponds with the presence of the pars recta of the proximal tubules, while no parts of the proximal tubule are in the inner zone of the external medulla.

The division of the kidney into cortex and medulla is also based on the anatomy of its vascular supply. After entering the hilus of the kidney, the renal artery divides into two sets of end-arteries, which progressively subdivide into further arteries, the

interlobar and the arcuate arteries. The interlobar arteries bend
over the bases of the pyramids, at the juction between cortex
and medulla, to form a series of incomplete arches, the arcuate
arteries. From these arteries there rise at right angles interlobular arteries which run radically towards the periphery of
the cortex. The interlobular arteries give off numerous short
branches, the afferent arterioles, each of which directly supplies
one glomerulus. From the glomerular capillaries, the blood is

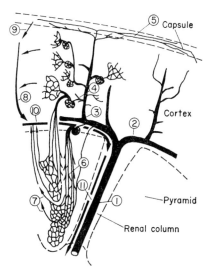

FIG. 2.2 Diagram showing blood supply of renal parenchyma,
based on work of Fourman and Moffat, Morison, and Trueta *et
al*. Veins indicated by arrows. (1) Interlobar artery; (2) Arcuate
artery; (3) Interlobular artery; (4) Intralobular artery; (5)
Capsular plexus; (6) Arteriolae rectae spuriae; (7) Venae rectae;
(8) Interlobular vein; (9) Stellate vein; (10) Arcuate vein; (11)
Interlobar vein (from Bell, Davidson & Scarborough, 1968).

carried by the efferent arterioles to the tubules. The vascular
supply of the tubules is essentially a portal one, the blood that
perfuses the peritubular capillaries having previously passed
through the glomerular capillary vessels (Fig. 2.2).

The vascular supply of the cortical nephrons differs from that
of the juxta-medullary nephrons. The efferent arterioles of the
cortical nephrons break up into a freely anastomosing network of
capillaries which envelope the convolutions of the proximal and

distal tubules, as well as the upper part of the ascending and descending thick limbs of the loop of Henle and of the collecting tubes. In the juxtamedullary zone of the human kidney some glomeruli have short and others long efferent arterioles. The short ones (about 7000) supply blood to the juxta-medullary parenchyma. The long efferent arterioles (about 180,000) descend into the medulla, where each one branches into two arteriolae rectae containing smooth muscles in their walls. It is suggested that the muscles of the medullary arterioles serve to ensure the adequacy of the circulation of the cortex rather than that of the medulla (Edwards, 1956). From these arterioles rise capillary vessels which follow the descending limb of the loop of Henle through the medulla and the papilla, turn at the bend of the loop, and return to reassemble into a venule which enters an interlobular vein close to its junction with an arcuate vein (Pitts, 1963). These capillaries, the *vasa recta*, are the only vessels carrying blood to the medulla. Despite their importance, there is little information as to their anatomy (Figs 2.3 and 2.4).

According to Moffat & Fourman (1963), who studied the renal blood vessels of several laboratory mammals and of man, the vasa recta vessels either end in capillary plexuses at various levels of the medulla or are unbranched vessels forming a plexus at the tip of the papilla. Plakke & Pfeiffer (1964) in their study used animals possessing widely different abilities to concentrate urine: the kangaroo rat (*Dipodomys*) the gerbil (*Meriones*), the opossum (*Didelphis*), the cat, the pig, the beaver (*Castor*) and the *Aplodontia*. Their view is that the 'vasa recta arise in leashes from the efferent arterioles of the juxta-medullary glomeruli and descend, many as unbranched vessels, in parallel bundles to break up into capillary plexuses at different levels of the medulla. These plexuses drain via ascending, parallel vessels into branches of the arcuate and interlobular veins.' They were, however, 'unable to find any true loops, such as those figured in many physiology texts and reports, and described in detail by Trueta (1948)' (Plakke & Pfeiffer, 1964).

Moffat & Fourman (1963) had shown that in the mammals examined by them the capillary plexuses that arise from the descending vasa recta differ in their arrangement, so that there is a dense peritubular network in the inner stripe of the outer zone, and a relatively sparse plexus in the outer stripe of the outer zone and in the inner medullary zone. This zonation, which was

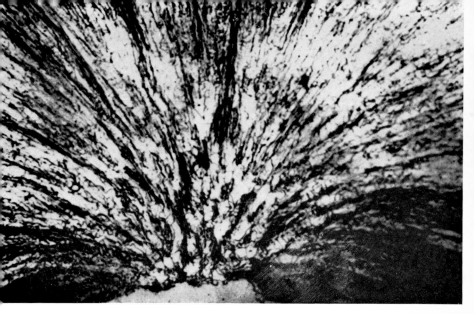

FIG. 2.3. Vasa recta and collecting ducts from *Aplodontia rufa* showing the openings of collecting ducts into the renal sinus (Nungesser & Pfeiffer, 1965).

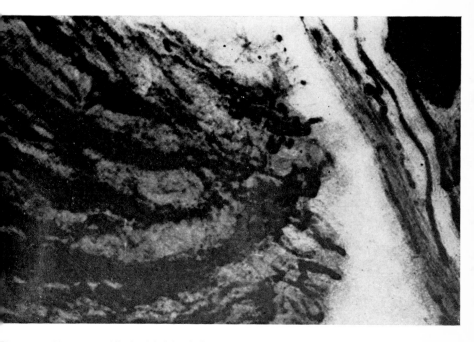

FIG. 2.4. Vasa recta filled with blood from the kidney of *Aplodontia rufa* (Nungesser & Pfeiffer, 1965).

(Facing p. 20)

observed also by Plakke & Pfeiffer (1964; 1965), exists, however,
only in the kidneys of mammals (cat, rat, kangaroo rat) which are
capable of producing a highly concentrated urine, whereas in the
pig, the beaver (Plakke & Pfeiffer, 1964) and the *Aplodontia*
(Pfeiffer *et al.*, 1960) there is no such zonation. In these animals

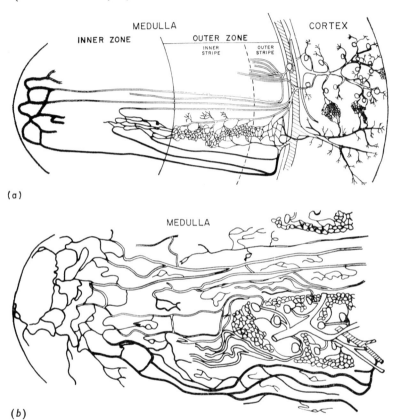

FIG. 2.5 (*a* and *b*). Diagrammatic representations of the vascular
bed of the kidneys of two mammals, the opossum (*a*) and the
beaver (*b*), showing the presence of zonation of the opossum (*a*)
and its absence in the beaver (*b*) (after Plakke & Pfeiffer, 1964).

the same type of plexus arises from each vas rectum whether in
the inner, middle or outer zone of the medulla and there are more
branches and anastomoses of vasa recta than in the species showing
zonation (Fig. 2.5). According to these authors, in most mammals

the zonation of medullary blood vessels is related to the zonation that results from the architecture of nephrons. For instance, in the *Aplodontia*, the beaver and the pig, there is no true inner zone of the medulla (Sperber, 1944; Pfeiffer *et al.*, 1960) and hence no zonation of nephrons. Whether these observations can be extended to the sloth, *Choloepus hoffmanni* Peter (Goffart & Nys, 1965) is not known.

The arrangement of the renal blood vessels, with capillaries as the only source of blood to the medulla, suggests at once that the blood flow to the two regions of the kidney must be very different (Weaver, McCarver & Swann, 1956). Until recently it was possible to measure the blood flow through the whole kidney only. Plethysmographic and flowmeter methods are among the techniques which have been used. They cannot, however, provide any information as to the flow through a specific part of the renal blood vessels, such as the capillary network of the vasa recta. To achieve this, three different methods have been used: one based on clearance and extraction of para-aminohippuric acid, another on the injection of dyes, the third on the rate of washout of injected isotopes.

The clearance of para-aminohippuric acid at low plasma concentrations, corrected for incomplete extraction, is conventionally used to estimate total renal plasma flow in the intact animal and man. In man and most mammals, the average value for the extraction ratio of para-aminohippuric acid is of the order of 0·91. In 1958 Reubi suggested that the incomplete extraction of para-aminohippuric acid was due to the fact that in the kidney there was a mixture of two flows; one, the clearing or cortical flow, from which para-aminohippuric acid is 100% extracted and the other, the non-clearing or medullary flow, from which no para-aminohippuric acid is extracted. According to Reubi's view, 91% of the plasma perfusing the kidney is completely cleared of para-aminohippuric acid; this represents the cortical flow which perfuses the proximal convolutions of both cortical and juxta-medullary nephrons. The remainder, from which no para-aminohippuric acid is removed, represents the medullary flow, which irrigates the loops of Henle, the collecting ducts and inert tissue. Reubi's assumption was experimentally confirmed by Pilkington, Binder, de Haas & Pitts (1965), who showed that during osmotic diuresis, following an intravenous infusion of a 20% mannitol solution, both the cortical and medullary flow and the total renal plasma flow increased, the medullary flow increasing proportionately more than the cortical flow. An intravenous infusion of acetylcholine (50–80 μmoles/min) had a similar effect, whereas an infusion of noradrenaline (3·8–9·0 μmoles/min) decreased the cortical and the total renal plasma flow, but did not affect the plasma flow of the medulla.

The blood flow (*BF*) of an organ can be calculated from its vascular volume (*VV*) and the mean circulation time (*t*) by the following equation:

$$BF = \frac{VV}{t}$$

The mean circulation time (*t*) through a tissue can be estimated from dilution curves of injected dye recorded at the end of the vascular bed (Nanninga, Swann & Schubert, 1962). This technique, which has been widely used for the estimation of blood flow through different tissues, was adapted by Kramer, Thurau & Deetjen (1960) and Thurau, Deetjen & Kramer (1960), in an attempt to estimate the circulation time within the vascular bed of the medulla itself. To do this, they placed, in an anaesthetized dog, a photocell and a source of light on opposite sides of the renal papilla. The dye (Evans blue or Cardiogreen) was injected into the renal artery. The vascular volume (*VV*) was calculated from the intravascular haematocrit value obtained from direct measurement (Ullrich, Pehling & Stöckle, 1961) and from the concentration of haemoglobin; O_2 saturation was determined photo-electrically as a mean value over the total length of the vasa recta. From such studies, Kramer and his collaborators estimated that the blood flow through the inner medulla represented about 1% of the total renal blood flow.

Whereas Kramer and his collaborators measured the blood flow through the medulla only, Barger (1966) developed a method of washout of isotopes which would give information as to the blood flow in the different regions of the organ. It was based on a technique which had been described and used for the study of myocardial blood flow (Herd, Hollenberg, Thoburn, Kopald & Barger, 1962), and is essentially an application of the Fick principle: when the blood that passes through an organ loses some constituent, then the quantity of the constituent lost per unit time is equal to the difference between the quantity entering

B

through the arterial blood in the same time and the quantity leaving through the venous blood. The American authors injected ^{85}krypton dissolved in a physiological solution into an artery of an anaesthetized dog and determined the venous rate of washout with the use of a scintillation counter. Whereas in the myocardium or any other tissue, the rate of disappearance of ^{85}krypton followed a simple exponential curve, in the kidney the situation was different. After the injection of ^{85}krypton, the renal pedicule was ligated and the kidney was extirpated and frozen immediately in an acetone–dry ice mixture. The frozen kidney was then sliced into 1 mm cross-sections which were placed in contact with X-ray film between plates at -50 °C. If the kidney was removed from the animal immediately after the injection of ^{85}Kr, radioactivity was present in the cortex, the blood vessels and the perirenal fat. If 15 seconds elapsed between the time at which ^{85}Kr had been injected and the kidney was removed, radioactivity was found also in the outer medulla. If, however, the kidney was removed 2 min after the injection of ^{85}Kr, the cortex was cleared of radioactivity, the bulk of it being in the medulla. Using this technique Thoburn, Kopald, Herd, Hollenberg, O'Marchoe & Barger (1963) estimated the rate of disappearance of the radioactivity which they found was distributed into four different exponential curves, one for the cortex, one for the outer-medulla, one for the inner-medulla and the last for the perirenal and hilar fat. From these data, they calculated that in the normal anaesthetized dog, the blood flow through the cortex averaged 400–500 ml./min/100 g tissue; in the outer-medulla 120–150 ml./min/100 g, and in the inner-medulla 12–20 ml./min/100 g only. Thus approximately 84% of the total blood flow through the kidney goes to the cortex, about 13% to the outer-medulla and about 3% to the inner-medulla (Barger, 1966).

As for lymphatic vessels, it would appear from the rather scanty literature on the subject that there is a greater lymphatic system in the renal cortex and a lesser one in the medulla where it follows the course of the vasa recta (Kaplan, Freidman & Kruger, 1942; Goodwin & Kaufman, 1956; Selkurt, 1963; Balics & Rényi-Vamos, 1967). More recent electronmicroscopy investigations have revealed, however, that the medulla has a rich network of lymph capillaries, whereas in the cortex the majority of the capillaries are blood capillaries (Rhodin, 1965). The results obtained by various

TABLE 2.1

Relation between thickness of renal cortex and medulla and urine concentration in mammals

	Cortex (mm)	External medulla (mm)	Internal medulla (mm)	Medulla (internal and external) (mm)	Ratio (int. med./cortex)	Maximum osmolar concentration of urine (m.-osmole/l.)	References
Beaver	7·0	14·0	0·0	14·0	0·0	600	O'Dell & Schmidt-Nielsen (1960)
Aplodontia	4·2	5·0	0·0	5·0	0·0	600	Nungesser et al. (1960); Dicker & Eggleton (1964)
Pig	20·0	7·5	6·5	14·0	0·3	1100	O'Dell & Schmidt-Nielsen (1960)
Rabbit	5·0	5·0	10·0	15·0	2·0	1500	O'Dell & Schmidt-Nielsen (1960)
Dog	7·0	6·0	11·0	17·0	1·6	2000	Ullrich et al. (1955)
Hamster	1·5	1·6	4·1	5·7	2·7	3000	Morel & Ginnebault (1961)
Dipodomys	1·0	1·2	3·8	5·0	3·8	5700	Schmidt-Nielsen (1964)
Psammomys	2·1	2·4	11·5	13·9	5·5	6000	Schmidt-Nielsen (1964)

authors on the volume, flow and composition of the lymph whether drained from the cortical or the hilar network are so contradictory that no opinion as to its role could be formulated. Recently, however, Santos-Martinez & Selkurt (1969) have attempted a re-appraisal of the problem. Using anaesthetized dogs they investigated the drainage of the lymph in the kidney with a view to determining if the renal lymph is in some way related to the counter-current system. They studied the hilar lymph-to-arterial plasma ratios of urea, sodium, potassium, creatinine, p-aminohippuric acid and osmolarity under conditions which either increased the lymph flow and osmotic pressure of the medulla or produced a washout of the electrolyte gradient. Their results suggest that the lymph drained from the cortex is mixed with that coming from the medulla and that the constituents of the medullary lymphatics which drain the lymph towards the juxta-medullary zone come into equilibrium with the vasa recta by a process of exchange diffusion. This lymph then joins the lymph drained from the cortex where an osmotic equilibrium with arterial blood is achieved (Henry, Keyl & Bell, 1969).

Transverse sections of kidneys of different animals show that the thickness of either the cortex or the medulla varies from species to species, but that for each species there seems to be approximately the same ratio between medulla and cortex. For instance, in *Dipodomys*, the kangaroo rat, the medulla is approximately five times thicker than the cortex, whereas in *Aplodontia rufa*, a sciuromorpha, the medulla and cortex have the same

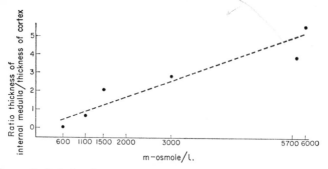

FIG. 2.6. Relation between urine concentration and ratio thickness of internal medulla/thickness of cortex of kidneys of some mammals. In abscissa the values (m-osmole/l.) are those referred to in Table 2.1.

thickness. Both animals, however, belong to the order Rodentia. But whereas the kangaroo rat is one of the mammals which has the greatest capability to conserve water, *Aplodontia* appears to be the least efficient in this respect (Pfeiffer *et al.*, 1960; Dicker & Eggleton, 1964*a*). Since the medulla contains most of the thin limbs of the loops of Henle, physiologists pointed out a possible correlation between the ability to concentrate urine and the length of the loop and especially of its thin segment. This had been suggested already by Peter (1909). Though the data on which Peter based his findings scarcely warranted his conclusion, it was supported by Crane (1927) who noted that hypertonic urine was formed only by the kidneys of mammals and of birds in which a thin segment was present. The thin segment of the loop of Henle is absent in reptiles and all lower forms of vertebrates. None of them can produce a urine which is more concentrated than their plasma or glomerular filtrate. In birds, though ill-developed, the thin segment is present but only in a small number of the animal's nephrons (d'Errico, 1907). In 1933, Burgess, Harvey & Marshall suggested that since the thin limb appeared to be the site of urinary concentration, it was there that the neurohypophysial hormones acted to promote water reabsorption, leading to urine concentration. Soon, however, the role of the thin limb as a site for urine concentration was rejected on the ground that the epithelium of this segment was too thin to perform significant osmotic work (Smith, 1951), though it had long been recognized that other very thin epithelia such as the frog's skin or fish gills (Smith, 1930; Bevelander, 1935) could perform remarkable amounts of work against osmotic gradients. Another reason for discarding the role of the thin limb of the loop of Henle in the process of urine concentration, was the finding by Walker *et al.* (1941) that in dehydrated rats in which the osmotic pressure of the urine was markedly higher than that of the plasma, micropuncture of the distal tubule revealed that the fluid in it which had just gone through the loop, was either hypotonic or at best iso-osmotic to the glomerular filtrate.

In 1944, Sperber published the results of his study on the kidneys of more than 140 species of mammals living in widely different surroundings. He found that without distinction of group mammals which live in a wet climate have a kidney characterized by the absence of a papilla. As the environment becomes less humid, the presence of a papilla becomes a feature of the kidney, and animals living in an arid habitat have a big papilla. For instance, *Ornythorhyncus*, a Monotreme living in a humid climate, has a kidney without papilla, whereas another monotreme, *Antechinomys*, living in an arid environment, has a kidney with a well-developed papilla. Among Rodentia, *Aplodontia*, which lives in a humid area of the American Pacific Northwest (Pfeiffer *et al.*, 1960), has no papilla, *Psammonys*, the so-called sand rat, which lives in a very arid area, has comparatively the biggest papilla. A similar division, between kidneys without and with a papilla can be found among chiroptera and primates according to whether they eat succulent or dried food. Recently Pfeiffer (1968) pointed out that the renal pelvis of mammals is different according to whether the animals can or cannot concentrate their urine. He described two types of pelvis. In type I, the pelvis is an uncompli-cated, slightly expanded ureteral ending, while type II is an exten-sive chamber whose wall is thrown into elaborate folds that reach deep into the renal medulla. Among mammals with a renal pelvis of type I are the *Aplodontia*, the beaver and the domestic pig. The kidneys of *Aplodontia* and beaver have a medulla without an inner zone and the pig has only a very small inner zone. In contrast to animals with a well-developed type II pelvis, those with type I renal pelvis are known not to be able to concentrate their urine well.

Though Sperber was the first to recognize the correlation between the ecology and the feeding habit of animals with the anatomy of their kidney, more recent studies have shown that some rodents which had been classified previously among animals which live in arid desert conditions are in fact 'moist' (Schmidt-Nielsen, 1964). For instance, though *Psammonys* is a desert rodent, its habitat is restricted to places where the vegetation has a high water content. The plants among which it nests are salt-loving plants, similar to the halophytes found at the edge of saline and brackish water all over the world. Some of these plants contain more than 800 milli-equivalents of NaCl per kg fresh plant, thus about twice the NaCl content of sea water (Schmidt-Nielsen, 1964). The sand rat eats great quantities of these plants, which contain between 80 and 90% water. The *Psammonys* can handle the salt quite readily. Its urine output averages 1·0 ml./h/g.b.w., containing up to 1900 m-equiv of Na, with a total osmotic con-centration of the order of 6000 m-osmole/l.

Though one would expect that rodents which thrive on dry food only without ever drinking would concentrate their urine even more than 'moist' rodents which eat succulent food containing appreciable amounts of water, this is not so. The kangaroo rat, *Dipodomys merriani* (Schmidt-Nielsen, Schmidt-Nielsen, Brokaw & Schneiderman, 1948) or the gerbil, *Gerbillus gerbillus* (Burns, 1956), eat dry seeds and other dry plant material, even when succulent plants are available. They do not drink water. The osmotic pressure of their urine is of the order of 5500 m-osmole/l. with a urine/plasma ratio of 14. The ratio between the size of the internal medulla and that of the kidney of *Dipodomys* is 0·6 (Morel & Guinebault, 1961), which is of the same order as that in *Psammonys*; the ability to concentrate urine is very similar in both.

Recently Schoen (1969) has studied three bovids from East Africa: the bushbuck, *Tragelaphus scriptus dama* from moist bushland, the Uganda kob, *Adenota kob thomasii* from dry savannah and the dikdik, *Rhyncotragus kirkii* from semi desert habitat, and found that when these animals were dehydrated to about 85% of their initial body weights, their urine output fell as follows: the bushbuck from 99·1 ± 8·4 to 69·7 ± 2·0, the kob from 46·4 ± 3·7 to 27·2 ± 1·5 and the dikdik from 10·9 ± 0·77 to 1·3 ± 0·04 ml/kg/day. Their urine concentration rose for the bushbuck from 936 ± 52 to 1369 ± 52, the kob from 1109 ± 16 to 1594 ± 11, and for the dikdik from 2235 ± 138 to 4762 ± 62 m-osmole/l. Measurements of the kidneys of the three species showed that the medulla occupied 31, 38 and 47% of the kidneys respectively. On the assumption that the volume of the medulla is a measure of the length of the loops of Henle, these results would suggest that the capacity to concentrate the urine is related to the aridity of the habitats of these tropical bovids.

Of interest are the observations made by Hummel (1963) on *Meriones Shawii Shawii* (Duvernoy), a North African desert rat, of the order of Rodentia; it feeds on a dry diet and like the gerbil can live without ever drinking (Schmidt-Nielsen, 1964). If given water by stomach tube it is unable to excrete it. When, however, it is fed a diet containing progressively more fresh vegetable, it will eventually be able to excrete water which has been orally administered, like any other rodent. Its water diuresis may then even exceed that of a white rat. This change in its ability to excrete urine follows a radical change in its renal haemodynamics: the blood flow through the renal medulla of *Meriones* fed on lettuce was found to be twice that in *Meriones* kept on a dry diet (Hummel, 1963).

Though the classification proposed by Sperber (1944) may have to be modified slightly there is a clear relation between the size of the renal medulla and the ability of the kidneys to concentrate their urine. And since the renal medulla, and especially its inner zone with the papilla, contains only thin limbs of the loops of Henle (called long loops by Sperber) there would appear to be a correlation between the number and length of the long loops and the ability of a kidney to concentrate its urine. For instance, whereas rodents like *Dipodomys*, *Psammonys* or *Gerbillus* which all have nephrons with long loops extending into the renal papilla, can concentrate their urine very well, another rodent, *Aplodontia rufa*, which has cortical nephrons only with very short loops that do not reach the medulla, cannot concentrate its urine (Pfeiffer *et al.*, 1960; Dicker & Eggleton, 1964*a*). Furthermore, in the kidneys of *Aplodontia* or of beaver there is no inner zone of the medulla, the entire medulla being homologous to the outer zone of species like the rat. Finally, it will be remembered that in the domestic pig, which can elaborate urine with a maximum osmotic pressure of 1100 m-osmole/l. only, the kidneys have only 3% of 'long looped nephrons' (Sperber, 1944) and a medulla with a very small inner zone (Morel & Guinnebault, 1961).

The question that arises now is whether those animals, which have evolved kidneys with a greater medulla and papilla, longer and more numerous long limbs of the loop of Henle, and a renal pelvis that develops chambers deep into the medulla, have acquired an anatomical configuration whose function is to concentrate, or whether these structures are an accident of nature without real physiological or functional meaning.

3
OSMOTIC PRESSURE GRADIENT IN THE KIDNEY

'*No kind of knowledge has ever sprung into being without an antecedent, but is inseparably connected with what was known before . . .*'

Payne (1897)

FILEHNE & BIBERFELD in 1902 and six years later Hirokawa (1908), using simple methods for estimating the freezing point of tissue samples, showed that the osmotic pressure of samples taken from the medulla of kidneys was higher than that of samples from the cortex. Having found that the osmotic pressure of the renal cortex was constant, and did not depend on the concentration of the urine excreted, Hirokawa stated: 'In contrast, the osmotic pressure of the renal medulla is extremely variable, and under normal conditions it is almost without exception higher than that of the cortex, and is the higher the more concentrated is the urine. . . . Our observations show unequivocally that the urine present in the medulla has a much higher osmotic pressure than the urine that is in the convoluted tubules of the renal cortex; therefore, the osmotic pressure of the urine increases considerably during the passage through the loops of Henle and collecting tubules. . . . An increase in the osmotic pressure of the urine in the renal medulla can obviously occur in two ways: either by a secretion of osmotically active material into the urine or by loss of water through reabsorption. In case the first possibility were the only correct one, the main secretory transport of urea and inorganic urine ingredients would not be performed in the convoluted tubules of the cortex, as assumed by the majority of physiologists in agreement with Bowman–Heidenhain's hypothesis, but by the loops of Henle and the collecting tubules in the medulla.' Hirokawa's findings and conclusions remained unnoticed for many years. Neither Smith nor his collaborators seem to have known them. In 1909 Grünwald published results according to which there was a greater concentration of chloride in the medulla than in the cortex. This was confirmed thirty years later by histo-chemical studies (Feyel & Vieillefosse, 1939), and by the work of Glimstedt (1942) and of Ljungberg (1947). Ljungberg cut sections 18·7 μ thick from a 3 mm core of rabbit's kidneys and estimated the chloride concentration in the sections. He found that the chloride concentration in such a column increases from cortex to medulla. In the cortex, the chloride concentration averaged 2·5 γ per section (or 142 mg/100 g tissue), whereas towards the apex of the medulla the sections contained 90 γ (1 g/100 g tissue). This figure exceeds the concentration of chloride in any other tissue. The progressive concentration of chloride in the medulla could not be attributed to the presence of urine in the collecting ducts because the total area occupied by the lumen of these ducts was less than 8% of the cross-section examined; and the chloride content of the medulla was unrelated to the chloride concentra-tion of the urine. Using various assumptions, Ljungberg (1947) estimated that the concentration of chloride in the cells of the proximal tubules was between 99 and 110 mg/100 g, whereas in the cells of the collecting ducts, the concentration of the anion was of the order of 2500 to 2700 mg/100 g, as against 360 mg/100 ml. in the plasma.

One of the features of evolution is the development by higher vertebrates of mechanisms capable of maintaining the extracellular fluid at a fairly constant composition. The osmolar concentration of extracellular fluid in mammals is usually of the order of 300 m-osmole/l. Opie (1949), however, found that considerably stronger solutions were required to prevent the swelling of slices of a number of isolated tissues. For instance, he found that solu-tions of sodium chloride isotonic with parenchymatous cells of liver or of kidney have twice the molar concentration of sodium chloride of blood plasma. Moreover, cells of the renal collecting tubules of mammals must be able to survive when in contact with anisotonic solutions. Considerations of this nature had led Siebeck (1912) to study the osmotic properties of the kidneys of frogs and Conway, Fitzgerald & McDougal (1946) those of mammals. Robinson (1950) reinvestigated the problem by incubating rats' kidney slices in media which preserved the cation

ratios of the extracellular fluid but differed in osmolar concentration and estimated the oxygen consumption of slices as well as
their water content. The results of these experiments showed that
oxygen consumption was more important than the osmotic
pressure of the external medium in maintaining the amount of
water in cells and that cells from the renal cortex of adult rats
were in osmotic equilibrium when immersed in media with an
osmotic pressure twice that of plasma. This was confirmed by
Dicker & Morris (unpublished) for slices of the renal cortex of
adult rats and guinea pigs. According to Robinson (1950) the
fact that cells from the renal cortex have an osmotic pressure of
about 600 m-osmole/l. can be explained only if energy derived
from respiration is used to expel water from the cells. This would
produce a steady state in which the higher internal osmotic
pressure would cause water to diffuse into the cells as fast as it is
pumped out. This interpretation, however, has been criticized
by Appelboom, Brodsky, Tuttle & Diamond (1958) and Swan &
Miller (1960) and subsequently revised by Robinson (1960).

In 1951, Wirz, Hargitay & Kuhn published the results of their
cryoscopic studies of renal tissue. Their technique was as follows:
rats were deprived of water for up to 48 hr. Under ether anaesthesia one kidney was removed and immediately dropped into
liquid air. The temperature of the frozen kidney was then allowed
slowly to increase until it reached − 10 °C when the organ was cut
into sections of 30 μ. Under very careful conditions of temperature
control, the thawing process was then followed and the loss of
optical birefringence determined under crossed Nicols. These
experiments showed that slices from the cortex were isotonic
with blood plasma, while slices taken more deeply from the renal
medulla were hypertonic to it. Starting from the junction between
the cortex and the medulla and going towards the papilla, there was
an approximately linear increase of the osmotic pressure. At the
tip of the papilla values of osmotic pressure between five to eight
times those of the plasma were observed. Moreover, within any
given cross-section, contents of all tubular formations had the
same osmotic pressure: the fluid in the limbs of the loops of Henle
had the same tonicity as the fluid in the neighbouring collecting
tubes (Figs. 3.1, 3.2, and 3.3). A few years later Bray (1960) using
a method similar to that of Wirz et al. (1951) studied rats' kidneys
removed either during antidiuresis or during a water diuresis. He

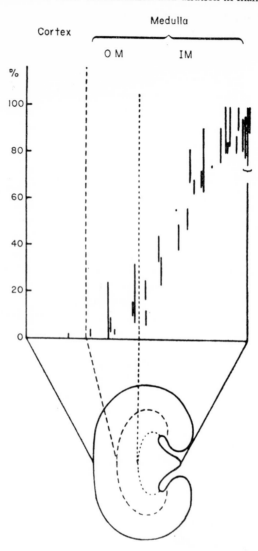

FIG. 3.1. Variation of the osmotic pressure as estimated from slices taken along the axis of the papilla. Values of the ordinate have been calculated as $= (\Delta_x - \Delta_{\text{isot}})/(\Delta_{\text{max}} - \Delta_{\text{isot}})$, the value 0 being that of plasma. It will be seen that all regions of the cortex are iso-osmotic with plasma, whereas those of the medulla are markedly hypertonic to plasma. (OM, outer medulla; IM, inner medulla)

(after Wirz *et al.*, 1951)

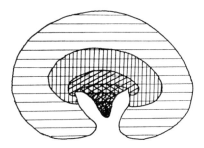

FIG. 3.2. Regions of equal osmotic pressure lie on concentric shells parallel to the zone boundary (from Wirz *et al.*, 1951).

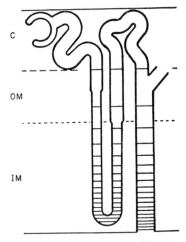

FIG. 3.3. Diagrammatic representation of the variation of osmotic pressure in a single nephron. The glomerulus, proximal and distal convoluted tubes are in the cortex and they have the same osmotic pressure. The osmotic pressure increases in limbs of the loop and the collecting duct as they are nearer to the papilla, in the inner medulla. C, cortex; OM, outer medulla; IM, inner medulla (after Wirz *et al.*, 1951).

confirmed that in hydropoenic animals the inner zone of the renal medulla had an osmotic pressure markedly greater than that of plasma, while in rats killed during water diuresis, the osmotic pressure of the inner medulla was slightly hypertonic to blood plasma or glomerular filtrate, with concentration values of about 500 m-osmole/l. Further, whereas slices from the renal cortex, from both hydropoenic and hydrated rats, were isotonic with blood plasma, those from the outer strip of the outer medulla were hypotonic.

Though Wirz *et al.* (1951) and Bray (1960) fully confirmed Hirokawa's prediction, results from cryoscopic studies of tissue samples must be assessed critically. With ordinary solutions of potassium or sodium chloride, as the temperature falls, ice will cease to separate out when the temperature and concentration of the solution have reached the eutectic point; the solution will then solidify as a whole. For a solution of potassium chloride, the eutectic condition is reached at a temperature of $-10 \cdot 8$ °C and a concentration of $3 \cdot 3$ M; for a solution of sodium chloride, at a temperature of $-21 \cdot 0$ °C and a concentration of $5 \cdot 2$ M. Protoplasm, of course, does not consist of a simple solution of either of these salts and the eutectic condition is likely to be reached at a somewhat higher temperature, and with less increase in concentration, partly owing to the presence of colloidal constituents (Bayliss, 1960). There is also the possibility of a diffusion of solutes occurring either during freezing or thawing of the preparation and of inevitable changes in protoplasm when ice crystals separate which may lead to an increase of the concentration of solutes within the cells (Berliner, Levinsky, Davidson & Eden, 1958) and the possibility of artefacts due to the size of crystals embedded in the cells (Bray, 1960).

Ullrich, Drenchkhahn & Jarausch (1955) using Opie's (1949) method determined the concentration of salt solutions with which tissue slices taken from various levels from a kidney of a dehydrated dog would be in equilibrium. The experiments confirmed the results of Opie (1949) and of Robinson (1950): slices from the cortex were in osmotic equilibrium in solutions of about 450 m-osmole/l.: i.e. in solutions slightly more concentrated than plasma; those from the medulla or the papilla, however, had a concentration of the order of 1800 to 2000 m-osmole/l. Of importance was the observation that, according to the concentration of the solutions in which the slices were immersed, cells showed either shrinking or swelling, suggesting that the intracellular fluid phase or compartment must have been involved in the ultimate process of osmotic stratification. As the slices taken from the tip of the papilla had an osmotic pressure similar to that of the urine collected before the dog was killed, and since the papilla consists mainly of collecting ducts, it was concluded that an osmotic equilibrium must obtain between the epithelium of these ducts and the intraluminal urine. Further, Ullrich et al. (1955), confirming Ljungberg's (1947) observations in the rabbit, observed that, in kidney slices from a dehydrated dog, the concentrations of sodium and of chloride increased with the osmotic pressure; i.e. the concentration of these two ions was greater in slices from the inner medulla than in those from the cortex. There was, however, no similar increase in the concentration of potassium. Sodium accounted alone for some 20% of the total osmotic pressure of slices from the renal papilla though its final concentration in the excreted urine was markedly lower. It was the concentration of urea which represented the most significant gradient, its concentration being about the same in the papilla as in the urine (500–700 mM/l.) (Ullrich & Jarausch, 1956) (Fig. 3.5).

When samples of kidney were taken from a dog in water diuresis, it was found that the osmotic gradient of the renal tissue was much less marked than during dehydration and that the greater the rate of urine flow the lower the osmotic gradient of the tissue. During water diuresis there was a gradient for sodium and chloride in the external zone of the medulla but none in the inner zone of the medulla. Finally in contrast with what had been found in dehydrated animals, in dogs undergoing a water diuresis the osmotic pressure of the urine was lower than that of the renal medulla (Ullrich, Drenchkhahn & Jarausch, 1955).

During an osmotic diuresis no osmotic pressure gradient could be observed in the renal slices, and the concentrations of sodium, chloride or urea were uniform. The papilla and the urine had comparatively low osmotic pressure values and the urea concentration, though low, was essentially the same in tissue slices and urine (Ullrich et al., 1955; Ullrich, Jarausch & Overbeck, 1955). Similar results were reported by Malvin & Wilde (1959) who suggested that high rates of flow through the loops of Henle were responsible for the washing out of elements producing an osmotic gradient.

Similar conclusions to those of Ullrich et al. (1955) were reached by Ruiz-Guinazu, Arrizurieta & Yelinek (1964) who estimated the sodium, chloride, urea and water content of kidney slices of dogs suffering from hydropoenia or undergoing a water diuresis. The concentration of the urine of the hydropoenic dogs varied between 1620 and 2340 m-osmole/l., that of hydrated dogs between 40 and 160 m-osmole/l. Whether the animals were dehydrated or not, the renal cortex had the same concentration of chloride and of sodium but in the outer medulla the concentration of these ions rose gradually until it reached its maximum in the inner medulla. The concentration of these ions in the medulla of dehydrated dogs was 30% higher than in dogs in water diuresis. The water content of the kidney slices was the same at all levels of the cortex, but increased in slices cut from the outer medulla, irrespective of the state of hydration of the animal. In the inner medulla, the water content rose towards the papilla during water diuresis but decreased during hydropoenia. As for urea, it showed no increase in concentration in the medulla during water diuresis, but a marked rise during hydropoenia.

The existence of a gradient of osmotic pressure in the kidney has since been demonstrated in other animals and in a variety of conditions. To mention a few only: Guinnebault & Morel (1957) observed a gradient for sodium, but not for potassium, in the renal tissue of rats which had been given a NaCl solution by stomach tube; Crabbe & Nichols (1959) found it in rats suffering from hydropoenia; an osmotic gradient for sodium during hydropoenia and its absence during osmotic diuresis was demonstrated in the dog (Malvin & Wilde, 1959); its existence was also confirmed in the kidneys of hamsters (Morel, Guinnebault & Amiel, 1960), rabbits (Morel & Guinnebault, 1961), sheep (Schmidt-Nielsen & O'Dell, 1959) and a variety of rodents (Schmidt-Nielsen & O'Dell, 1960). In contrast, in animals such as the beaver, the domestic pig, *Aplodontia rufa* or birds which do not concentrate their urine well (Table 3.1), little or no renal osmotic gradient has been observed (House, Pfeiffer & Braun, 1963). For instance, in roosters a small increase in sodium and chloride concentrations was noted from cortex to medulla during dehydration and salt-loading, but the difference between cortex and medulla for the two ions was not greater than 14·0 and 17·7 m-equiv/l. for sodium and 15·2 and 19.1 m-equiv/l. tissue water for chloride. The concentration of potassium was the same in the cortex and the medulla (Skadhauge & Schmidt-Nielsen, 1967). The small osmotic pressure gradient found in the kidneys of dehydrated or salt-loaded birds is related to their poor ability to concentrate their urine and agrees with the observations that their urine osmolarity

TABLE 3.1

Comparison between urine and plasma osmolarity at the time of maximum urine concentration following administration of vasopressin, in two rodents: *Aplodontia rufa* and rabbit

Animal	Plasma (m-osmole/l.)	Urine (m-osmole/l.)	U/P
Aplodontia	292	430	1·47
	295	420	1·42
	290	460	1·59
	300	500	1·67
		Average	1·53
Rabbit	288	890	3·09
	295	1015	3·44
	288	910	3·16
	290	925	3·19
		Average	3·22

does not usually exceed 550–600 m-osmole/l. with a ratio U_{osm}/P_{osm} of about 1·4–1·5 (Owen & Robinson, 1964; Dicker & Haslam, 1966; Skadhauge & Schmidt-Nielsen, 1967).

Since the osmotic pressure had been determined on kidney slices which contained besides urine, tubular cells, blood and lymphatic vessels and interstitial tissues, the meaning of the results remained somewhat obscure until the osmotic pressure of each part could be measured separately. The first to attempt this was Wirz (1953) who used the kidneys of hamsters. The renal papilla of the hamster is easily accessible. It contains collecting tubules along with a few thin limbs of loops of Henle and their accompanying vasa recta. But whereas the loops and collecting tubes are well below the surface of the papilla, the vasa recta are seen running on its surface, where they appear as capillaries. Using the technique of micropuncture, Wirz withdrew blood from the capillary vessels of the papilla and estimated its osmotic pressure, which he then compared with that of urine. He found that, according to the rate of urine flow, the freezing point of urine varied between − 0·56 and − 0·94 °C. Blood taken simultaneously from the renal papilla had the same freezing point as the urine; the difference between samples of urine and blood taken simultaneously being less than 0·05 °C. Blood from the systemic circulation had a freezing point of between −0·52 and −0·59 °C. Thus, it was shown not only that blood from the vasa recta had the same freezing point value as the urine excreted, but that blood in the capillaries of the medulla of the kidney has an osmotic pressure three to four times that of the systemic blood.

These results were confirmed by Gottschalk & Mylle (1958, 1959) and by Gottschalk, Lassiter, Mylle, Ullrich, Schmidt-Neilsen, O'Dell & Pehling (1963) on adult rats, hamsters (*Mesocricetus auratus*), kangaroo rats (*Dipodomys spectabilis*) and *Psammonys obesus*. Under sodium pentobarbital (35 mg/kg) anaesthesia, the animals were given a priming dose of 25 μc of urea-^{14}C and inulin (50 mg/kg), followed by a constant intravenous infusion of inulin (2 mg/min/kg). After allowing about 1 hr for equilibration, approximately 0·15 μl. of fluid was collected by micropuncture from the bend of loops of Henle at the tip of the exposed renal papilla. In each case the lumen of the loop had been blocked distally to the site of the puncture by the injection of a droplet of mineral oil. Before and after each collection, urine from a nearby collecting duct and blood from the vasa recta were collected. All samples were divided under oil and their osmolality determined by the microcryoscopic method of Ramsay (1949) and Ramsay & Brown (1955), while inulin was estimated spectrophotometrically and urea-^{14}C in a windowless flow proportional counter (Lassiter, Gottschalk & Mylle, 1960, 1961). These experiments showed that the osmolalities of the fluid collected from the bend of the loop of Henle and of the urine in the collecting tube were essentially the same. The osmotic pressure of the fluid in the loop of Henle was made up of 64% of sodium and attendant anions and of 19% urea. In the collecting duct, however, urea was the major constituent, while the concentration of sodium was low. From inulin estimations, it was calculated that about 9% of the amount of water filtered by the glomeruli reached the tip of the loops at a time when 0·9% of water only was in the final urine. Furthermore, fluids collected from the bend of loops of Henle, from collecting ducts and from vasa recta at the same level in the kidney had an osmotic pressure essentially similar, but markedly greater than that of the systemic blood (Gottschalk & Mylle, 1959).

In 1941, Walker and his co-workers had shown that, whereas the fluid in the proximal tubule of rats was iso-osmotic with the glomerular ultrafiltrate, the fluid in the distal tubule was *hypotonic*

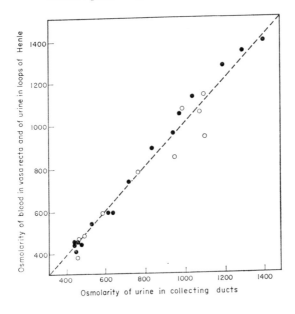

FIG. 3.4. Relation between the osmotic pressure of urine in the loops of Henle and in the collecting ducts and the osmotic pressure of blood in the vasa recta. Urine was collected from the loops of Henle and from the collecting ducts and blood from the vasa recta by micropuncture technique in hamsters, kangaroo-rats and *Psammonys*. Note the similarity of the osmotic pressure in urine and blood. Abscissa and ordinate: m.osmole/l. Abscissa: urine in the collecting ducts, ●, urine from loops of Henle; O, blood from vasa recta (adapted from Gottschalk and Mylle, 1959).

to plasma. Admittedly they managed the micropuncture and the collection of fluid from the distal tubule on three occasions only, and only in two of these samples did they find an osmotic pressure below that of plasma. Wirz in 1956 repeating the experiments of Walker *et al.* (1941) did effectively show that the osmotic pressure of the fluid collected from the early part of the distal convoluted tubule of the rat is *always* lower than that of plasma. During hydropoenia, however, the hypotonic fluid becomes isotonic as it reaches the collecting tubes, though the urine excreted may be

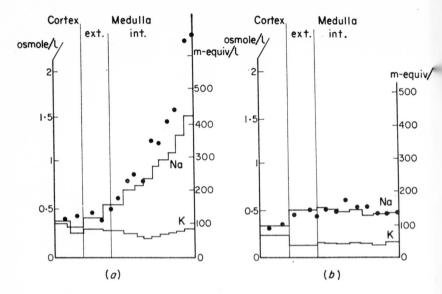

FIG. 3.5. Osmotic gradient and tissue electrolytes of the kidney of the dog, (*a*) in the hydropoenic and (*b*) in the hydrated animal. ● = value of osmotic pressure as estimated in slices taken from different regions of the kidney.

several times more concentrated than the plasma. The elaboration of a concentrated urine, therefore, can be achieved in the collecting tubes only. In contrast, during water diuresis, the urine remains hypotonic to the plasma along the whole length of the distal tubule, and since the osmotic pressure of the urine is much lower than that collected from the distal tubule, the final dilution of the urine must likewise take place in the collecting tubes (Wirz, 1956).

The events occurring as the urine goes down the collecting tubes were studied by Hilger, Klümper & Ullrich (1958) using the method of multiple site catheterization of the collecting tubes evolved by Jarausch & Ullrich (1957). Collecting tubes of hamster were cannulated with microcatheters at varying points along their length. Samples were collected simultaneously from sites near the junction between cortex and medulla and nearer the end of the tubules in the region of the papilla at 2·7 and 1·3 mm from the tip of the papilla. Inulin was used as a reference substance. The average inulin concentration and osmolarity of the tubular fluid collected at 2·7 mm was 1603 mg/100 ml. and 572 m-osmole/l., while the average inulin and osmolar concentration of the fluid collected at 1·3 mm from the tip was 2412 mg/100 ml. and 633 m-osmole/l. respectively. Thus, between the upper and lower points of catheterization the inulin concentration had increased 1·5-fold while the total osmolar concentration had increased by 1·1 time only. The increased concentration of inulin could have been achieved by water reabsorption only. As for the concentration of sodium and potassium of the fluid collected from the upper and lower sites from the collecting tubes, the potassium concentration increased by an amount similar to that of inulin while that of sodium fell from an average of 174 to 96 m-equiv/l. (Table 3.2).

TABLE 3.2

Results of micropuncture of collecting tubes in kidneys of hamsters

Distance from tip of papilla (mm)		Inulin (mg/100 ml.)		Osmolarity (m-osmole/l.)		Sodium (m-eqiv/l.)		Potassium (m-eqiv/l.)	
Us	Ls	Us	Ls	Us	Ls	Us	Ls	Us	Ls
2·7 (34)	1·3 (34)	1603 (33)	2412 (33)	572 (33)	633 (33)	174 (26)	96 (26)	32 (25)	51 (25)
		Ls/Us 1·5		Ls/Us 1·1		Ls/Us 0·6		Ls/Us 1·6	

The data collated from those published by Hilger, Klümper & Ullrich (1958) are given as averages. In brackets, number of experiments or estimations. Us =upper site of micropuncture, Ls =lower site of micropuncture. The distance between the two sites was 1·4 mm.

These experiments then showed that there is a steady rate of water reabsorption along the collecting tubes accompanied by an increase in the osmotic pressure. Sodium is reabsorbed at a higher rate than water, while potassium does not appear to be affected. Subsequently, Klümper, Ullrich & Hilger (1958) showed that, in contrast to sodium, urea appeared to be reabsorbed together with water from the collecting tubes. Its back diffusion is in all likelihood passive.

The experiments, whether involving cryoscopic estimations of tissue slices, osmotic equilibration of tissue fluid with external solutions, or the analysis of fluids collected by micropuncture from loops of Henle, vasa recta and collecting tubes, demonstrate without exception that in the kidneys of mammals elaborating a hypertonic urine there is a gradient of osmotic pressure which reaches its maximum in the tip of the papilla. But whereas all segments of the nephrons, at a determined depth, have the same osmolarity, they do not necessarily have the same fluid composition. For instance as shown by Schmidt-Nielsen, Ullrich, O'Dell, Pehling, Gottschalk, Lassiter & Mylle (1960) the ratio between the concentration of sodium in the fluid of the proximal tube and in plasma is 0·97 in the hydropoenic rat, but 0·75 only in the rat during osmotic diuresis. In the tip of the papilla, the ratio between the concentration of sodium in the fluid of the loop and that in the blood plasma increases with the osmotic pressure, whereas in the early part of the distal convoluted tubule it falls below unity. Since the ratio U/P for sodium in the distal tubule reaches a value of 0·62 during oliguria and of 0·25 during osmotic diuresis, while the U_{osm}/P_{osm} ratio at the same site is equal to 0·75, in either oliguria or polyuria, it would appear that sodium is actively reabsorbed along the ascending limb of the loop of Henle without any corresponding amount of water. Similarly, Lassiter, Gottschalk & Mylle (1960) and Gottschalk, Lassiter, Mylle, Ullrich, Schmidt-Nielsen, O'Dell & Pehling (1963) showed that in the desert rat there is addition of urea to the fluid of the descending limb of the loop, whereas the cells of the ascending limb appear to be impermeable to both urea and water.

It is clear then that the elaboration of the composition of the urine and the changes of its osmotic pressure are two relatively independent processes and that to understand the ultimate mechanism of urine concentration and/or dilution they must be investigated separately.

4

CHEMICAL ELABORATION OF THE URINE

THE osmotic pressure gradient of the concentrating kidney is made up of solutes among which sodium, potassium and urea play a major role. Since there are parts of the kidney in which the tubular fluid has more sodium than in others, and since the excreted urine contains less sodium than urea, it is important to review the renal tubular mechanisms involved in the elaboration of the urine. The treatment of sodium, potassium and urea by the different parts of the nephron will be discussed in that order.

There is now overwhelming evidence to support the observations by Wearn & Richards (1924) on amphibians and of Walker and his associates (1941) on mammals that the fluid in the proximal tubule is iso-osmotic with the glomerular filtrate, and that while in the proximal convolutions it is reduced in volume. From estimations made by micropuncture it has been calculated that about 45% of the filtered water is reabsorbed in the surface convolutions of the proximal tubule in the dog (Bennet, Clapp & Berliner, 1967). As two thirds only of the proximal tubule are accessible to direct investigation, this is in fair agreement with previous estimations according to which about 70–80% of the glomerular filtrate was reabsorbed iso-osmotically. The absence of changes of the osmotic pressure of the fluid in the proximal tubule could be attributed either to the primary movement of water followed by NaCl, or alternatively to the movement of NaCl followed by water. This has been investigated using the technique of 'stopped flow microperfusion' of a single proximal tubule of the kidney of *Necturus*. In this technique a fluid of known composition is introduced into a proximal tubule whose lumen is blocked at both ends with oil. Windhager, Whittembury, Oken, Schatzmann & Solomon (1959) perfused the proximal tubule of *Necturus* with solutions iso-osmotic with plasma, but containing various amounts of NaCl, the total osmolar concentration of 187 m-osmole/l. being made up by addition of mannitol when required. The concentrations of NaCl varied from 50 to 100 m-equiv/l. If transport of water initiated that of NaCl, net water flux should be independent of NaCl tubular concentration; conversely if water movement were dependent upon NaCl concentration, a relationship should obtain between the two variables. From changes in the concentration of mannitol in the proximal tubule and of mannitol injected, the water reabsorption could be calculated as

$$\phi^w = 1 - \frac{Man_0}{Man_i} \times 100$$

where ϕ^w = water flux; Man_0 = concentration of mannitol injected into the tubule and Man_i = mannitol concentration in the collected perfusate. It was found that for NaCl concentration of 100 m-equiv/l. in the tubule, the percentage of water absorbed was of the order of 26, and for NaCl concentration of 50 m-equiv/l. it was − 9, the negative sign indicating a net water movement into the tubule. Thus it could be shown that there is a close relation between water reabsorption and NaCl concentration, and that water flux is nil when net solute flux is zero. It could be demonstrated, further, that net movement of Na takes place up an electrochemical potential gradient, indicating active transport of this ion, while movement of water from or into the tubule is a passive transport which can be accounted for quantitatively in terms of osmotic activity arising from net solute movement (Maude, Shehadeh & Solomon, 1966).

(a) Sodium

The reabsorption of sodium in the proximal convoluted tubule raises several points such as the relation of sodium transport to the electrochemical forces and to the movement of water, the adjustment between the rates of sodium reabsorption and of glomerular filtration, and the factors regulating proximal tubular sodium transfer.

An active process will apply to any ion movement that takes place against electrochemical driving forces operating across a single cell boundary. It excludes transfer by passive diffusion and by bulk movement of fluid, but includes carrier mediated transport down an electrochemical potential gradient if it is energy consuming and if it proceeds at a rate in excess of that expected from the electrochemical driving forces (Giebisch & Windhager, 1964). The movement of sodium out of the lumen of any part of the nephron proceeds against an electrical potential gradient: the whole length of the tubular lumen has been found to be negative with respect to the peritubular fluid (Solomon, 1957; Whittembury & Windhager, 1961; Clapp, Rector & Seldin, 1962; Kashgarian, Stoeckle, Gottschalk & Ullrich, 1963; Burg, Isaacson, Grantham & Orloff, 1968). With respect to the interstitial tissue, the lumen of the proximal tubule is some -20 to -25 mV negative, that of the descending limb of the loop of Henle -3 mV, that of the ascending limb about -11 mV, that of the distal tube -49 mV, and that of the collecting tube some -14 mV (Gertz, 1962, 1963; Giebisch & Windhager, 1964). These findings have been confirmed by experiments in which the electrical potential gradient was abolished by application of an opposing electromotive force. In these conditions, the electrical current that can be measured across a segment of a nephron is of a magnitude equivalent to the net movement of sodium ions across similar tubular segments (Eigler, 1961; Windhager & Giebisch, 1961).

Tubular sodium reabsorption is correlated with oxygen consumption (Deetjen & Kramer, 1960; Kramer & Deetjen, 1961). When the stoicheiometric relationship between the Na and O_2 was measured, it was found that about 20–30 equiv of sodium were reabsorbed per mole of oxygen used (Torelli, Milla, Faelli & Constantini, 1966). This is in good agreement with measurements of oxygen consumption and sodium transport in other epithelial membranes.

Water reabsorption in the proximal tubule is osmotically coupled with the transport of sodium. From the calculated amounts of sodium chloride reabsorbed per unit time, the tubular surface area and the permeability coefficients, it was estimated that in the rat a transtubular osmotic gradient of 23 m-osmole/l. must be postulated if water movement were induced as a result of osmotic pressure. It is known, however, from cryoscopic studies of tubular fluid and of plasma that no osmotic pressure gradient exists along the proximal tubule (Wirz, 1956). To explain this apparent

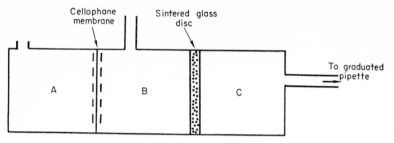

FIG. 4.1. Schematic representation of the model proposed by Curran & Macintosh. The solution in A was stirred by a stream of air and that in C by means of a magnetic stirrer. Solution in B was not stirred and the exit tube to B was sealed during the experiment.

When identical solutions were placed in all three compartments there was no detectable net volume flow in either direction. Net flow of water from A to C was observed when the solute concentration in A was less than that in B, but greater than in C. Thus between A and C there appeared to be a net movement of water against a water concentration gradient.

discrepancy Curran & McIntosh (1962) and Ullrich & Rumrich (1963) have suggested somewhat complicated models consisting of a non-expansible compartment of which one side is a semi-permeable membrane and the other is freely permeable, the compartment being itself situated between two others accessible for fluid sampling (Fig. 4.1). In this system the creation by sodium transport of a concentration gradient across the semipermeable membrane would involve the passive transfer of water, which in turn would raise the hydrostatic pressure in the non-expansible compartment. The increased hydrostatic pressure would lead to hydraulic flow into the peritubular fluid compartment across the membrane which is assumed to be equally permeable to solutes and water, and does not therefore allow the development of an osmotic pressure gradient across it. Though there is no proof that this model works in the same way as the proximal tubule, the peritubular cell membrane and the basement membrane of the proximal part of the nephron may qualify as structures with the proposed differences in permeability (Giebisch & Windhager, 1964). An interesting development of Curran & McIntosh's model is that formulated by Diamond (1964) and Whitlock & Wheeler

(1964) which would explain how solute-linked water can flow against an osmotic gradient (Skadhauge, 1969).

As for chloride, it has been known for some time, that contrary to sodium, its concentration in the fluid of the proximal tubule may exceed that in plasma (Lichtfield & Bott, 1962; Kashgarian et al., 1963) and that the extent of this rise is dependent on the degree of acidification of the fluid. For several decades it had been assumed that the reabsorption of chloride from the fluid in the proximal tube is passive. Abramow, Burg & Orloff (1967), however, showed that though ouabain depresses the peritubular transmembrane potential in the kidney of Necturus, it failed to decrease the exchange rate of chloride in the renal tubule cells of the rabbit. The view that the flux of sodium represents transtubular transport of NaCl may therefore have to be modified (Zadunaisky & De Fisch, 1964).

Why does the reabsorption of sodium or sodium chloride in the proximal tubule proceed only to some 80% of the amount filtered? Two explanations have been suggested. First, since the reabsorption of sodium chloride is decreased in the presence of poorly reabsorbable solutes such as mannitol or urea, there may be a limiting concentration gradient across the pars recta of the proximal tubule (Pitts, 1959; 1963). Second, since there is no evidence of a concentration gradient for sodium along the part of the proximal tubule accessible to micropuncture, it has been suggested that the remainder of the tubule may have different characteristics of transport and permeability which might favour the development of such a gradient, such as a weaker pump or a pump working in the presence of higher permeability to sodium (Giebisch & Windhager, 1964).

Another question arises from the observation that the same percentage of the filtered sodium is reabsorbed in the proximal tubule irrespective of whether the increased amount of sodium comes from an increased concentration of sodium in the plasma or from the combination of increased filtration rate and increased plasma sodium concentration (Selkurt, 1954; Pitts, 1959; Giebisch, Klose & Windhager, 1964). Several hypotheses have been advanced to explain this. Walker et al. (1941) suggested that the amount of water and of sodium reabsorbed in each segment of the proximal tubule is proportional to the amount that reaches it; thus in their view progressively smaller amounts of sodium would be reabsorbed along the tubule. Kelman (1962) has tried to draw an analogy between the pattern of reabsorption in this part of the nephron and the kinetics of a catalytic flow reactor system. Such a system is characterized by the fact that the rate of reaction for fixed concentrations of substrate is an increasing function of the rate of flow. Thus at low glomerular filtration rate, the incomplete mixing of the fluid in the lumen would result in a reduced concentration at the site of the catalytic reaction which would lead to a radial concentration gradient of the substrate. At higher glomerular filtration rate such effect would be minimized and the radial concentration for sodium would be dissipated. Later Kelman (1965) calculated the extent to which sodium reabsorption would proceed when related to the length of the proximal tubule and showed that his results were in fair agreement with those expected from the theory of kinetics of catalytic flow reactor. Unfortunately most of the length of the tubule in which a more precise discrimination of the pattern of sodium reabsorption could be achieved is inaccessible to micropuncture. Leyssac (1963) investigated the problem more directly. He observed the time needed for the occlusion of the renal artery to produce a complete collapse of the lumen of the proximal tubule and used this as a measure of the rate at which sodium is reabsorbed in the tubule. The occlusion time was compared with the rate of filtration immediately before the clamping of the renal artery. These experiments led to two important findings: first, the reabsorption of fluid, and hence of sodium, continued after cessation of filtration; second, when related to the filtration rate immediately before ligation of the renal pedicle, there was a direct proportionality between reabsorption and pre-existent formation of filtrate. Thus, in these experiments changes in the rate of flow as a consequence of changes in glomerular filtrate rate could not be seen to play a role. Thurau (1966) suggested that the reabsorption of sodium in the proximal tubule was controlled by a feedback mechanism within the macula densa. Instead of estimating the time needed for complete occlusion of the proximal tubule, Thurau injected by micropuncture some lissamine green into an early part of the proximal tubule. By following its passage along the nephron by serial microphotographs, he measured the inner diameter of the tubule. He then injected in the early part of the distal tubule solutions of NaCl of various concentrations. Since the macula densa is located up-stream from the site of the puncture, the injection was directed towards it (Fig. 4.2). In normal conditions the concentration of sodium chloride in the tubule in the region of the macula densa is of the order of 40 m-equiv/l. Thurau injected solutions of NaCl of 75, 150 and 300 m-equiv/l. When solutions of 150 to 300 m-equiv/l. reached the macula densa, the proximal tubule collapsed. This was interpreted as an indication that the glomerular filtration had ceased. In these experiments, glomerular filtration was interrupted only in those nephrons which had been injected; filtration was never affected in adjacent ones. The duration between onset of the injection and the collapse of the proximal tubule was 15–20 sec; the collapsed tubule reopened approximately 60 sec after the end of the injection. When choline was substituted for sodium or when sodium-free mannitol solutions were injected towards the segment of the macula densa, glomerular filtration was not affected. Thurau then repeated these experiments on two groups of rats, one kept on a Na-free diet to increase the concentration of renin in the granular cells of the macula densa and the other in which the macula densa had been depleted of renin by unilateral nephrectomy four weeks before the experiment (Thurau & Schnermann, 1965; Cortney, Nagel & Thurau, 1966; Schnermann, Nagel & Thurau, 1966). Only in rats with a high content of renin in the kidneys did an increased concentration of sodium produce cessation of filtration followed by collapse of the proximal tubule. From these experiments, Thurau concluded first, that within a single nephron unit, 'a functional connection exists between the macula densa and the glomerulus, the character of which is an inverse relation between sodium concentration in the tubular fluid near the macula densa and filtration rate (sodium feedback mechanism)'. Second, that the strict localization of this reaction to the single nephron unit and the dependence on the renin content of the granular cells suggest that this reaction is mediated by the function of the juxtaglomerular apparatus (Thurau, 1966).

Yet another hypothesis proposed by Gertz (1963), Gertz, Mangos, Braun & Pagel (1965), Rector, Brunner & Seldin (1966) and by Brunner, Rector & Seldin (1966) is that the rate of sodium reabsorption is influenced by changes in the geometry of the lumen of the proximal tubule. This was confirmed recently by Wiederholt, Hierholzer, Windhager & Giebisch (1967) who studied

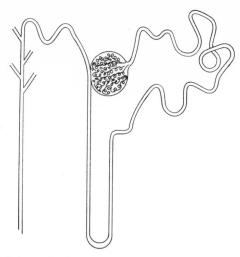

FIG. 4.2. Schematic drawing of the anatomical arrangement of a single nephron showing how the glomerulus comes into contact with the ascending limb of the loop of Henle.

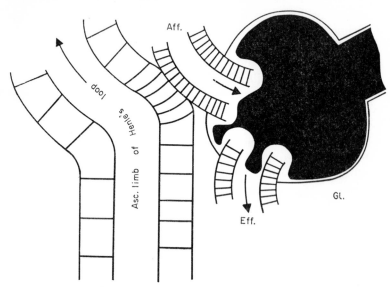

FIG. 4.3. Schematic representation of the point of contact between the ascending limb of the loop of Henle and the vascular pole of the glomerulus. The macula densa cells are those cells of the limb which are against the afferent arteriole.

Aff. = afferent glomerular arteriole; Eff. = efferent glomerular arteriole; Gl. = glomerulus.

the effect of alterations in tubular geometry brought about by different rates of volume flow on fluid reabsorption. For this purpose single proximal tubules of rat kidneys were perfused with Ringer solutions at different rates of flow. They found that the rate of fluid reabsorption was related to changes of diameter of the lumen of proximal tubules and estimated mean linear velocity of flow of the perfusate. They suggested that net transport of sodium in the proximal tubule changed in proportion to the cross-sectional area of the lumen of the tubule.

Finally, the possibility that the reabsorption of sodium by the proximal tubule may be affected by hormones of the adrenal cortex, should not be overlooked (Wright, Knox, Howards & Berliner, 1969).

There is also a marked reabsorption of sodium across the epithelium of the loop of Henle. This process is important as this part of the nephron is actually concerned in the elaboration of a concentrated urine. The transfer of sodium across the epithelium of the loop is accompanied by the establishment of a significant concentration gradient for sodium. From a comparison of the concentrations of inulin and of sodium found at the tip of the loops of Henle and in the early part of the distal tubule, it was shown that it is in the ascending limb that these gradients are established and that active sodium reabsorption takes place. Since from micropuncture studies as well as from cryoscopic investigations it is known that the fluid in the early part of the distal convoluted tube is hypo-osmotic to plasma (Wirz, 1956; Gottschalk & Mylle, 1958; Gottschalk et al., 1963) it follows that the ascending limb must be less permeable to water than the proximal tubule. Since the loops of Henle are located in the renal medulla, it is conceivable that the medullary blood flow plays a part in the establishment of the concentration gradient against which sodium has to be pumped. The rate of medullary blood flow may vary markedly (Thurau, Deetjen & Kramer, 1960). There is frequently an increase in the rate of sodium reabsorption along the loop when there is an increase of the renal medullary blood flow: this is due to a decrease of the transtubular concentration gradient as a result of the increase in the rate of medullary blood flow with the accompanying washout of medullary sodium. An example of this is what happens during an osmotic diuresis, when a decrease of the amount of sodium reabsorbed normally by the proximal tubules is compensated by an enhanced transport of sodium out of the loop of Henle (Windhager & Giebisch, 1961), accompanied by an increase of blood flow and a decrease of osmotic pressure gradient (Malvin & Wilde, 1959; Thurau *et al.*, 1960). The existence of a mechanism by which the loops compensate variations in the rate of sodium reabsorption in the proximal tubule can also be illustrated by experiments on single proximal tubules during water diuresis in the dog. In the absence of antidiuretic hormone, sodium reabsorption was found to be significantly inhabited (Clapp, Watson & Berliner, 1963). In some of these experiments, only about a third of the amount of sodium normally reabsorbed in the proximal tubule was removed from the lumen. Since no appreciable amount of the excess sodium present in the proximal tubule was found in the urine, it was concluded that it must have been reabsorbed along the loop of Henle. Thus an enhanced excretion of sodium, which might have occurred as the result of a diminished reabsorption in the proximal tubule, was prevented by an adaptive process in the loop of Henle. Similarly, when intravenous injections of hypertonic sodium chloride solutions are given in rats, the reabsorption of sodium along the loop of Henle increases to such an extent that the total amount of sodium reabsorbed remains fairly constant over a wide range of salt loading (Giebisch *et al.*, 1964). Evidence that the transport system for sodium in the loop of Henle is not easily saturated can be gained also from the fact that the concentration gradient for this ion is not abolished or even decreased under conditions of salt loading (Giebisch *et al.*, 1964). Similar conclusions regarding the capacity of the loop of Henle for transport of sodium have been reached from clearance studies in man (Eisner, Porush, Goldstein & Levitt, 1962; Goldberg & McCurdy, 1963). It is interesting to note, however, that the adaptive mechanism of the loop of Henle does not appear to exist in the dog or the rabbit. In these animals, during an osmotic diuresis produced by intravenous infusions of mannitol (Wesson & Anslow, 1948), of urea (Mudge, Foulkes & Gilman, 1949) or of hypertonic sodium chloride solutions Selkurt, 1954) the excretion of sodium was of such a magnitude that it could be explained only by the fact that the capacity for reabsorption in the loop of Henle had been exceeded.

The ability of the loop of Henle to adapt its capacity to reabsorb sodium might be dependent on its length. This, however, does not appear to be the case. Following the mathematical analysis of the relation between pressure and flow in the proximal tubule, a model has been derived in which these hydrodynamic factors were integrated. The function of the model was tested over a wide range of glomerular filtration rates, and the results confirm that the rate of sodium reabsorption by the proximal tubule is controlled by a negative feedback mechanism which accounts for the continued delivery of sodium and water in the distal part of the nephron, irrespective of variations in the physical characteristics of individual nephrons such as the length of loops of Henle (Bossert & Schwartz, 1967).

In contrast with the adaptivity of the loops of Henle, the distal tubules are not able to deal easily with increments of sodium chloride, since their capacity for transport is limited. Gertz (1962) showed the differences in the treatment of Na in the proximal and the distal convoluted tubes in the rat kidney in the following way: proximal and distal tubules of a rat kidney were punctured and injected with coloured castor oil. The column of oil was then broken with injections of NaCl solutions and the puncture site was sealed off. The rate at which the volume of the injected solutions changed was recorded through sequence photomicrography; these changes allowed the estimation of transtubular liquid flow per unit area and unit time. In proximal tubules, the time required for 50% of the injected solution to be reabsorbed was 9·8 sec, in the distal tubule it was 40 sec, indicating that the rate of Na reabsorption was four times slower in the distal than in the proximal tubule.

In the living animal, there is a close relationship between the volume of extracellular fluid phase and the rate of Na excretion by the kidneys. It is only quite recently that this relationship has been studied quantitatively. Brenner & Berliner (1969) have investigated the mechanism by which an expansion of the extracellular fluid volume produced by intravenous infusions of isotonic NaCl solution into rats and dogs is followed by an enhanced renal excretion of sodium. Using the "recollection micropuncture technique" they showed that the increased excretion of sodium was not due to an enhanced glomerular filtration or to an reduced level of circulating mineral corticoid hormones, but was produced by an inhibition of sodium reabsorption by the proximal convoluted tubule. Furthermore, they showed that the proximal tubule is able

c

to adjust fractional reabsorption of sodium in response not only to large, but also to small variations of the extracellular fluid volume.

A depression of the reabsorption of sodium in the proximal tubule will lead to an increment of sodium delivered first to the loop of Henle and subsequently to the distal convoluted tubule and collecting duct. Since neither Schnermann (1968) nor Morgan & Berliner (1959) were able to detect an inhibition of sodium transport by the loop of Henle following intravenous infusions of large quantities of isotonic NaCl solutions and since it would appear (Hayslett, Kashgarian & Epstein, 1967; Landwehr, Klose & Giebisch, 1967) that there is no depression of the sodium reabsorption by the distal tubule, it follows that the natriuretic response to the expansion of extracellular fluid phase is the consequence of a depressed sodium reabsorption in the proximal tubule and at some more distal portion of the nephron such as the cortical collecting tubule and/or the collecting duct.

Finally, the collecting duct is also a site where sodium is reabsorbed. It is along this segment that the steepest concentration gradients for sodium can be observed. It is particularly marked under conditions of sodium depletion, when the urine is almost sodium free. But, however steep the gradient, the contribution of this part of the nephron to the overall amount of sodium reabsorped is small: 1 or 2%, as compared with 86–90% for the proximal tubule and loop of Henle combined. Of interest is the fact that the concentration gradient which normally exists along the collecting duct can be either abolished by the administration of diuretic drugs or even reversed by administration of large doses of vasopressin (Ullrich & Marsh, 1963). Since there is evidence of a bidirectional movement of sodium across the tubular epithelium (Chinard & Enns, 1955) and since vasopressin would appear to act by increasing the permeability of the epithelium of the collecting duct to water, a similar increase of permeability to sodium may explain the natriuretic response to the antidiuretic hormone, which has been postulated for certain mammals.

(b) Potassium

Normally far less potassium is excreted in the urine than is filtered by the glomeruli. Since, however, there are situations in which potassium excretion exceeds the amount filtered, it must be concluded that the epithelium of the tubules is capable of both secretion and reabsorption of this ion (Mudge, *et al.*, 1948). Since from clearance experiments (Berliner, 1961) and from micropuncture studies of the rat nephron (Malnic, Klose & Giebisch, 1966*a*, *b*) it would appear that potassium is completely reabsorbed by the proximal tubule, Berliner (1961) postulated that potassium in the urine must have been secreted in the distal tubule. Berliner's view is also supported by results from experiments in which it was shown that after administration of radioactive potassium to a rabbit or to man the specific activity of the urinary potassium before complete isotope equilibration, was similar to that of renal venous potassium, but different from that of arterial blood plasma from which the potassium had filtered (Morel, 1955; Blake, Davies, Emery & Wade, 1956; Goldman, Yallow & Grossman, 1963).

The role played by the various segments of the renal tubule in the excretion of potassium has only recently been investigated in single nephrons. These studies, however, have been mainly confined to the rat; they ought to be repeated on other species. Rats fed either on a normal or on a low potassium diet, or which had been treated with kaliuretic drugs, were used. The concentration of potassium in the proximal tubule was compared with inulin and potassium concentrations in the plasma. The general pattern of handling of potassium by the proximal tubule was fairly similar in the three groups of rats, in spite of a variation in urinary potassium excretion which varied from a mean of 3% of the filtered potassium in animals on a low potassium diet to 150% of the filtered potassium in the others (Giebisch & Windhager, (1964) Although the concentration gradients which were established across the proximal tubular epithelium were small, extensive fluid reabsorption accounted for the reabsorption of the whole of the potassium filtered along the proximal tubule. The movement of potassium was active since it occurred against an eletrochemical gradient (Malnic *et al.*, 1966*a*, *b*).

The concentration of potassium in the fluid collected from the tip of the loops of Henle exceeds that in plasma. Since little or no potassium is found in the early part of the distal tubule, it must be assumed that potassium is secreted into the lumen of the descending limb while it is reabsorbed in the ascending limb.

In microperfusion experiments of single distal tubules of kidneys from *Necturus* with a potassium-free solution, it was found that potassium from the bathing fluid enters the tubule and reaches a concentration approximately the same as that of the extracellular fluid.

Little is known about potassium reabsorption along the collecting duct. The fact that with respect to the interstitial tissue the electropotential difference of the collecting duct is smaller than that of the distal tubule may be favourable to the hypothesis of an outward movement of this ion. It would thus appear that even in circumstances in which the amount of potassium in the urine greatly exceeds that which has been filtered most of it is reabsorbed by the proximal tubule and the ascending limb of the loop of Henle, while the excreted potassium is of predominantly secretory origin (Potter, 1946, Berliner, 1961).

(c) Urea

The other important component of urine is urea. It plays an important part in the production of a concentrated urine in mammals. In the frog, in contrast to mammals, urea appears to be actively secreted by the kidneys (Walker & Hudson, 1937*b*). As shown by Schmidt-Nielsen & Shrauger (1963), a high arginase activity is found in the kidney of the adult frog, *Rana catesbeiana*; urea is actively transported across the wall of the tubule, though formation of urea in the tubular cells is insignificant. In mammals, the renal tubules have on the whole a low permeability to urea, a curious feature since urea is distributed throughout the body water and penetrates most other living cells with ease. From comparative physiology, it is interesting to note that the respiratory epithelium in the elasmobranch, in contrast with that of bony fishes, is so impermeable to urea that it is present in blood in concentrations of 2000 to 2500 mg/100 ml. According to Smith (1951) in cartilagenous fishes and in frogs, urea is secreted by the tubules, but not in *Necturus*. It is passively reabsorbed by the tubules in the elasmobranch.

According to Clapp (1966) the concentration of urea rises above that in the plasma very early in the proximal tubule of rats, after which about half of the filtered urea diffuses out of the proximal tubule (Lassiter, Gottschalk & Mylle, 1961; Ullrich, Schmidt-Nielsen, O'Dell, Pehling, Gottschalk, Lassiter & Mylle, 1963). In the early part of the distal tubule, the amount of urea exceeds that in the glomerular filtrate, which suggests that urea has been added to the tubular fluid during its passage through the loop of Henle. With a urea concentration of 10 mM in the plasma, Schmidt-Nielsen (1962) found that at the end of the proximal tubule the concentration of urea amounted to 15 mM and in the early distal convolution to 65 mM. From analyses of kidney slices, she found that the osmotic pressure of the outer zone of the renal medulla of rats in antidiuresis was twice that of blood with a urea concentration 13 times that of plasma. Further down in the medulla, where the long loops of Henle are found, the concentration of urea was still higher. Results from micropuncture studies of the bend of the loop in the hamster papilla suggest that urea must have diffused into the lumen of the descending limb because the amount of urea present exceeded the amount filtered (Lassiter et al., 1961). During the passage of urine along the distal tubule, the actual amount of urea remains fairly constant, though its concentration is increased to about 190 mM, i.e. 19 to 20 times that of plasma, through water reabsorption. This agrees entirely with Bennet, et al. (1967) findings that in the dog about 45% of the filtered water is reabsorbed in the surface convolutions of the proximal tubule, 20% in the long loop of Henle, 10% in the distal tubule and 20% in the collecting ducts. Thus, it would appear that urea movements are largely, if not entirely, passive (Koike & Kellog, 1963; Lassiter, Mylle & Gottschalk, 1964).

The question is then how does urea accumulate in the renal papilla? It has been shown by microcatheterization of the collecting ducts in the hamster that about one third of the amount of urea leaves the collecting ducts (Klümper et al., 1958). If this is so, it may be that this is the source of urea in the renal medulla (Schmidt-Nielsen, 1962). According to Berliner et al. (1958) urea leaves the collecting tubes by passive diffusion, but from recent studies by Clapp (1966) it would appear that in protein-depleted rats urea may be actively reabsorbed from the collecting tubes. From the end of the distal tubules where urea concentration is of the order of 190 to 200 mM, down to the end of 2/3 of the length of the ducts, there is approximately a six-fold increase in the concentration of urea bringing it up to some 1140–1200 mM, by the time it reaches the zone permeable to urea. This six-fold increase in concentration of urea in the upper part of the collecting ducts is due to water reabsorption (Schmidt-Nielsen, 1962). It is in the lower third of the collecting ducts that urea diffuses back since the average concentration of urea in the lower part of the duct is 900 mM only. The hypothesis of a zone permeable to urea has some anatomical support, since in the kangaroo rat the wall of the collecting tube changes from cuboidal to flattened epithelium near the tip of the papilla (Schmidt-Nielsen, 1962).

Why does the urea remain in the medulla? Why does it not diffuse out? House *et al.* (1963) have suggested that the looped vasa recta are responsible for the trapping of urea in the medulla. More recently, Pfeiffer (1968) found a correlation between the concentration of urea in the renal medulla of mammals and their type of pelvis. According to this author, mammals with type II pelvis, with specialized fornices and secondary pyramids, have a much higher concentration of urea in their papilla than do those without them. This anatomical view is supported by the experiments of Gertz, Schmidt-Nielsen & Pagel (1966) who showed by per-fusing the rat pelvis that urea was added to the tissue of the papilla from the pelvis while water exchanges freely between pelvic urine and papilla.

It is possible now to summarize how nephrons elaborate the chemical composition of the urine. Starting with the entry of the glomerular filtrate into the proximal convoluted tube, there is an iso-osmotic reduction of the amount of fluid due primarily to an active reabsorption of sodium together with a passive reabsorption of water. Potassium is almost entirely reabsorbed (Berliner, 1961; Malnic *et al.*, 1966a). As the fluid runs down the descending limb of the loop of Henle, both urea and potassium enter into its lumen producing a high concentration of these solutes in the loop. At the same time some water may leave the lumen. In the loop itself the concentration of urea is at its highest. As the electrical gradient between the lumen and interstitial fluid at this site is small, there is no clear evidence of a transfer of sodium. In the ascending limb sodium is reabsorbed actively and so is potassium but the wall of the limb does not appear to be very permeable to either urea or water. The active reabsorption of sodium in the ascending limb is responsible for the hypotonicity of the fluid in the early distal convoluted tube. In this part of the nephron, potassium is secreted, while sodium is reabsorbed. Finally, in the collecting duct, while some sodium is reabsorbed, potassium may be both reabsorbed and secreted. As for urea, it diffuses out of the lumen of the duct in its lower third part, near the papilla. The final chemical composition of the excreted urine represents, then, the results of a complicated handling of its main constituents, some being transported actively, while others diffuse passively. It is in the light of its composition at the different stages during its journey along the nephron, and the formation of osmotic pressure gradients in some parts of the renal tubules, that the mechanism of concentration and/or dilution must be examined.

Addendum: Since there is good evidence to suggest that the proximal tubule cells of the mammalian nephron provide energy for the active transport of Na by oxidation mechanism, and that those portions of the nephron located in the medulla derive energy from aerobic and anaerobic glycolysis, the question is to what extent does oxidative and glycolytic metabolism contribute to Na reabsorption in the different parts of the nephron? Weinstein & Klose (1969) using micropuncture techniques in anaesthetized rats in which the renal arteries were infused with potassium cyanide and iodoacetamide showed that whereas cyanide acts by inhibiting Na reabsorption in the proximal tubule (without affecting the distal portions of the nephron) iodoacetamide inhibited Na and water reabsorption in all tubular segments, with the exception of the proximal convoluted tubule. These results would therefore indicate that the transport of Na in the proximal tubule depends upon metabolic energy available from the electron transport system which does not require glycolysis, whereas some or all other portions of the nephron require glycolysis for quantitative reabsorption of Na and water. Thus it would appear that there are different sources of energy for the reabsorption of the glomerular filtrate according to the portion of the nephron considered: the proximal tubule depending on oxidative metabolism, whereas the loop of Henle, the distal convoluted tubule and the collecting duct depend mostly upon glycolytic metabolism.

5

THE SINGLE EFFECT AND ITS MULTIPLICATION IN A HAIRPIN COUNTERCURRENT SYSTEM

'I often say that when you can measure what you are speaking about, and express it in numbers, you know something about it; but when you cannot express it in numbers, your knowledge is of a meagre and unsatisfactory kind; it may be the beginning of knowledge, but you have scarcely in your thoughts advanced to the stage of science, whatever the matter may be'.

William Thomson (1824–1907)

IT is now generally accepted that in mammals urine is concentrated through the operation of a countercurrent mechanism in the renal medulla, and that it is the countercurrent mechanism that is responsible functionally for osmotic stratification of the medulla. Though the overall course of events seems to be clear, the mechanism whereby the osmotic gradient is established and maintained needs critical appraisal.

Martin & Kuhn (1941*a*, *b*) and Kuhn & Martin (1941) published several papers on the 'multiplication' process as applied to the separation from mixtures of gases and of racemic compounds, which were followed by a paper by Kuhn & Ryffel (1942) in which the authors suggested that the process of multiplication by countercurrent might be applied to the kidney as a model to produce a concentration gradient. It was, however, not before 1951 that Hargitay & Kuhn introduced, as an 'exercise in physiological speculation', the concept of a 'hairpin countercurrent multiplier system' and published a theoretical analysis of it.

The principle of countercurrent has been known and applied in industry for many years. In its simplest form it can be illustrated by a jacketed tube such as a laboratory distillation column. Hot air enters the top of the tube and cold air is introduced through the bottom of the jacket; the direction of flow in the tube is opposite to that in the jacket, hence the term countercurrent. Heat will, of course, move across the wall separating the tube from the jacket thus penetrating into the cold compartment but heat will tend to be retained at the top of the system, while the temperature at the bottom will be only slightly higher than that of the incoming stream of cold air. The result of this arrangement is a large gradient of temperature between the two ends of the apparatus but only a very small difference in temperature across the tube at any given level. The efficiency of exchange will depend on the rate of flow: the slower the flow, the greater the time for equilibration between the opposite currents.

There are numerous examples of the principle of the countercurrent, especially with the aim of conserving heat, being used by animals. As early as 1876 Bernard had drawn attention to the arrangement between the warm arterial blood and the cooler venous blood forming a countercurrent. Venae comitantes accompanying the larger peripheral arteries have been described in man (Bazett, Love, Newton, Eisenberg, Day & Forster, 1948) and Bargeton, Durand, Mensch-Duchene & Decaud (1958) showed experimentally that the temperature of the arterial blood in the arm may be lowered by several degrees when the hand is cooled, but that there is a corresponding rise in the temperature of the venous blood returning to the heart. Systems of arteries and veins can thus work as heat exchangers. Another example is the arrangement of the pampiniform plexus of veins around the internal spermatic artery, which acting as a countercurrent exchanger helps in the maintenance within the scrotum of a temperature compatible with spermatogenesis. Other instances are provided by the whale and some aquatic birds. The whale is a warm-blooded homeothermic mammal that lives in arctic seas. Loss of body heat from the surface of extensively vascularized fins and flappers, appears to be prevented by the vascular arrangement of large arteries carrying warm blood suspended within a ring of cooler blood running in thin-walled veins. These concentric vessels act as a countercurrent heat exchanger which prevents the dissipation of heat peripherally and allows its conservation centrally (Scholander & Schevill, 1955). Similar arrangements exist in some warm-blooded aquatic birds which stand with their feet in cold water for prolonged periods: the arterial blood loses its heat and is cool by the time it reaches the feet, whereas the venous blood is warmed up and reaches a temperature of 37 °C as it gets into the body (Scholander, 1957, 1958; Metz, 1959).

The efficiency of the countercurrent system is increased when the countercurrent flow consists of a single tube that bends back upon itself, forming two limbs that are in close contact. This 'hairpin countercurrent system' has found its natural use in certain deep-sea fishes. In these animals the pressure of the gas in the systemic blood vessels is in equilibrium, through the epithelium of the gills, with that of the sea, which in turn is in equilibrium with the pressure in the air. The pressure of gas in the blood going to the so-called 'red gland' of the swim bladder, however, is much greater, as it must be the same as that in the swim bladder. The blood supply of the gland is through a *rete mirabile* which consists of closely intermingled capillaries running parallel to each other and to which afferent and efferent branches are connected by a hairpin bend. This system works as a very efficient countercurrent diffusion exchanger which can produce a steep tension gradient in excess of 100 atm of oxygen within the swim bladder by avoiding the loss of oxygen through outgoing blood (Scholander, 1954). Finally, the anatomical orientation of the nephron structures within the medulla provides the kidney of mammals with a battery of hairpin countercurrent systems arranged more or less in parallel: the descending and ascending limbs of the loops of Henle constitute one such system, and the branches of the vasa recta another. The problem in the kidney, however, is not that of heat conservation but that of a multiplier. As Hargitay & Kuhn (1951) put it: the kidney is faced with the problem of forming urine of an osmotic pressure of 70 atm from a plasma filtrate with an osmotic pressure of 7 atm only. This, they suggest, could be achieved if, in the kidney, there were a mechanism in which a *small* pressure acting on a semipermeable membrane were able to transform a solution of weak concentration into that of a higher concentration. Such a mechanism would be an application of a more general principle of multiplication defined previously by Kuhn & Martin (1941), and restated by Hargitay & Kuhn in 1951, which says that 'a high multiplication of a single effect can be produced in an elongated system in which there is a shift of the relative concentration of the order of $1 + d$ (single effect) across a transverse plane, under steady conditions.'

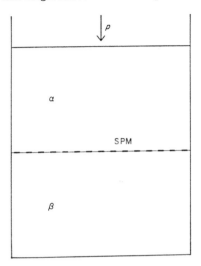

FIG. 5.1. Schematic representation of the single effect. Compartments α and β are filled with the same solution. SPM: semi-permeable membrane. p: hydrostatic pressure exerted on compartment α.

The single effect can be illustrated as follows: a vessel filled with a solution is divided into two equal compartments α and β by a semipermeable membrane, so that the same hydrostatic and osmotic pressures exist on both sides of the membrane (Fig. 5.1). If a pressure p is now exerted on the compartment α, some water will be forced through the semipermeable membrane which will result in an increase of the osmotic pressure in α with a corresponding dilution of the solution of β. As the pressure p is constant the passage of water through the semipermeable membrane will stop eventually and there will be a state of equilibrium which can be represented by

$$\Delta P = p = \Delta c \cdot RT \qquad (5.1)$$

in which p is the effective hydrostatic pressure, ΔP the difference between the osmotic pressure P in compartments α and β, Δc the corresponding difference in the concentration of the solutions in α and β, R the gas constant and T the absolute temperature. Since at the outset the volume v of α and β is the same let it be represented by v_0. Assuming that the initial amount of solute in α and β is n moles, then the initial concentration C_0 on either side of the semipermeable membrane will be $C_0 = n/V_0$ and the corresponding osmotic pressure will be $P_0 = RT \cdot C_0$. As a result of the action of the hydrostatic pressure p, a certain volume of water (Δv) will be pushed through the semipermeable membrane and the concentration in compartments α and β will change from C_0 to C_1 and C_2 respectively. Thus:

$$C_1 = \frac{1}{1 - (\Delta v/v_0)} C_0 \quad \text{and} \quad C_2 = \frac{1}{1 + (\Delta v/v_0)} C_0 \qquad (5.2)$$

When equilibrium is reached, the difference between the osmotic pressure in the compartments will be

$$\Delta P = (C_1 - C_2) \cdot RT = p \qquad (5.3)$$

From (5.3) p can be calculated as:

$$p = 2P_0 \cdot \frac{\Delta v/v_0}{1 - (\Delta v/v_0)^2} \qquad (5.4)$$

or by expressing $\Delta v/v_0$ in terms of concentrations C_0 and C_1:

$$p = RT \cdot \frac{C_1 - C_0}{1 - (C_0/2C_1)} \qquad (5.5)$$

and

$$p = \frac{P_1 - P_0}{1 - (P_0/2P_1)} \qquad (5.6)$$

The value of the osmotic pressure in α can be calculated as

$$P_1 = \frac{p + P_0 + \sqrt{(p^2 + P_0^2)}}{2} \qquad (5.7)$$

and that in β as;

$$P_2 = \frac{P_0 - p + \sqrt{(p^2 + P_0^2)}}{2} \qquad (5.8)$$

and since p/P_0 is very small, and the hydrostatic pressure is much smaller than the initial osmotic pressure of the solution,

$$P_1 \sim P_0 + \frac{p}{2} \quad \text{(approximately)} \qquad (5.7a)$$

and

$$P_2 \sim P_0 - \frac{p}{2} \quad \text{(approximately)} \qquad (5.8a)$$

Since, in this system, the osmotic pressure cannot increase beyond the value given in eqn (5.7a), when a state of equilibration has been reached the concentration in α and β will be that produced by the so-called 'single effect'. According to the general principle, however (Kuhn & Martin, 1941), this 'single effect', in which the changes in osmotic pressure are in a simple relation to hydrostatic pressure, can then be multiplied many times.

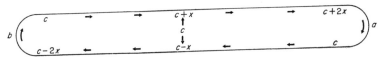

FIG. 5.2. Experimental model. For explanation see text below.

Consider an elongated vessel a–b containing a solution of concentration c, and let a force field (electric, magnetic or gravitational, etc.) be applied perpendicularly to its long axis with a strength just enough to produce and maintain between the upper and the lower part of the vessel a *small* displacement of the concentration of the order of $2x$ (single effect). Henceforth, there will be the formation of two layers with concentrations $c + x$ and $c - x$, respectively. If now the content of the vessel is brought into a slow motion, the layers of higher concentration and of lower concentration will gradually at the turning point tend to become equal again. At these points, the force field can again produce a displacement of the concentrations of the order of $2x$, in such a way that the layer of a concentration $c + x$, when reaching the upper part of the end a of the tube, will have a concentration $c + 2x$ while that in the lower part will be equal to c. As a result of a continuous motion, this process will repeat itself in such a way that at both ends the solution will have concentrations of $c + 3x$, $c + 4x$, ... $c + nx$, and $c - 3x$, $c - 4x$, ... $c - nx$, respectively. Eventually there will be a steady state during which there will be at one end a of the tube a strongly concentrated solution, whereas at the other end b, the solution will be very diluted. The difference between the concentrations at a and b will amount to $2nx$ in which the multiplication factor n will be approximately dependent on the ratio between the length and the width of the tube (Hargitay, Kuhn & Wirz, 1951). This was demonstrated in a model in which a tube ab filled with a solution of an osmotic pressure of 43 mm Hg was divided into two equal compartments by a semipermeable membrane. A hydrostatic pressure p of 65 mm Hg was applied on the upper compartment which, by forcing water out of it, increased its osmotic pressure to 93 mm Hg (single effect). After $8\frac{1}{2}$ days, the concentration of the solution measured at one end a of the model had an osmotic pressure of 185 mm Hg, thus demonstrating that the multiplication of a single effect had produced an increase of 142 mm Hg (Hargitay *et al.*, 1951).

Turning now to a 'hairpin countercurrent' system, consider a tube divided longitudinally into two equal compartments α and β, by a semipermeable membrane SPM (Fig. 5.3). At one end the two newly formed compartments α and β are linked together by a thin capillary tube K, while at the other end are fixed an inlet tube T_1 leading to α and an outlet tube T_2 coming from β. The entire

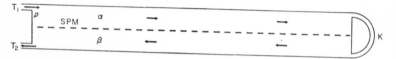

FIG. 5.3. Schematic representation of a hairpin countercurrent system. The solution enters by T_1, runs along α and leaves the system by T_2. K: thin capillary tubing. SPM: semipermeable membrane dividing the tube into two compartments α and β.

tube is filled with a dilute solution of salt and a small hydrostatic pressure p is applied at T_1 so as to produce a current flowing from T_1, through K, towards T_2, the solution then flows along a hairpin countercurrent. The diameter of the capillary tubing, K, is such that the difference of hydrostatic pressure which exists for each point along the tube is lost as the liquid flows through it. In this way the hydrostatic pressure p will produce a 'single effect'; i.e. the concentration of the solution in α and β will change in relation to its osmotic pressure, as expressed in eqns (5.7) and (5.7a). The solution which arrives at the hairpin bend will be a solution which has been concentrated; and since the 'single-effect' has operated all along the length of α, by the time the solution reaches the bend of the tube, its concentration will be greater than that resulting solely from one 'single effect'. It will have been multiplied. The solution entering β will have the same concentration as that of the solution α at the point of entry into capillary tube K.

This is illustrated in Fig. 5.4. The membrane separating the two limbs is permeable to water only, and the driving force is a hydro-

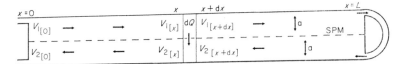

FIG. 5.4. Schematic representation of the multiplication of a single effect in a hairpin countercurrent system. For explanation see text.
The length of the limb is χ to L, so that T_1 of the model represented in Fig. 5.3 is $\chi = 0$. The solution enters the system with a velocity $V_{1[0]}$ and leaves it with a velocity $V_{2[0]}$. SPM: semipermeable membrane.

static pressure gradient between the two limbs. Filtration of water through the semipermeable membrane results in an increasing osmotic concentration of the fluid remaining in the descending limb, which reaches its maximum at the bend of the loop: the fluid flowing in the returning or ascending limb will be progressively diluted by the water that has come through the semipermeable membrane. Finally, in the steady state the osmolality of the fluid flowing out of the loop will be the same as that which entered it.

The mathematical analysis of this countercurrent multiplication operation has been worked out by Hargitay & Kuhn (1951). Consider a countercurrent apparatus in which the length of the limb will be from x to L, so that T_1 of the above model becomes $x = 0$. The cross-sectional area of the fluid stratum in both limbs is given as a, the length of the semipermeable membrane (SPM) as 1, the velocity of the incoming current is $V_{1[0]}$ and that of the outgoing fluid as $V_{2[0]}$. The velocity of the flow at any fixed point x will be $(V_{[1]})_x$ in one limb and $(V_{[2]})_x$ in the other. Since the solution enters the system by $x_{[1]} = 0$ and flows out by $x_{[2]} = 0$, it follows that

$$a \cdot V_{1[0]} = -a \cdot V_{2[0]} \quad \text{or} \quad V_{1[0]} = -V_{2[0]} \quad (5.9)$$

The pressure that drives the water through the membrane will be

$$\Delta p = p - [P_1(x) - P_2(x)] \quad (5.10)$$

where p is the hydrostatic pressure, $P_1(x)$ and $P_2(x)$ the osmotic pressure of the solution in both limbs as determined at a point x. The amount of water Q which will leave at the point x over the distance dx, each second, can be calculated as:

$$\left(\frac{dQ}{dt}\right)_x = y \cdot \Delta p \cdot dx = y[p - P_1(x) + P_2(x)]dx \qquad (5.11)$$

in which y is a proportionality factor which depends on the structure and thickness of the membrane, the viscosity and under certain conditions, the concentration of the solution, and can therefore be measured experimentally.

In other words eqn (5.11) means that the hydrostatic pressure p and the difference between the osmotic pressure $(P_1 - P_2)$ on both sides of the semipermeable membrane must be equivalent if they are to act as a driving force for water transport through the membrane (SPM). In practice, such an equivalence will obtain only if there is no concentration gradient in the solution on either side of the membrane.

In the limb T_1 (Fig. 5.3 and Fig. 5.4), the volume of liquid $a.(V_1)_x$ which will move each second from x to dx, will be equal to $a.(V_1)_{x+dx}$.

The volume of liquid $a(V_1)_x$ flowing through the cross-section at x is equal to the volume $a(V_1)_x + dx$ flowing through the cross-section at $x + dx$ together with the volume which flows through the membrane between x and $x + dx$. A similar argument applies to $a(V_2)_x$. Hence, remembering that V_2 is negative,

$$a \cdot (V_1)_x = a(V_1)_{x+dx} + y[p - P_1(x) + P_2(x)]dx \qquad (5.12a)$$

and

$$a \cdot (V_2)_x = a(V_2)_{x+dx} - y[p - P_1(x) + P_2(x)]dx \qquad (5.12b)$$

from which it follows that

$$\left(\frac{dV_1}{dx}\right)_x = -\left(\frac{dV_2}{dx}\right)_x \qquad (5.13)$$

Bearing in mind the condition expressed in eqn (5.9) for all values of x,

$$(V_1)_x = -(V_2)_x \qquad (5.14)$$

In a steady state of this system in which water can only pass from one limb into the other, there will, of course, be no changes in the concentrations in either limb. Thus for any point along the limb:

$$a \cdot V_{1[0]} \cdot C_{1[0]} = a(V_1)_x \cdot C_1(x) = -a(V_2)_x C_2(x) = -a \ V_{2[0]} \ C_{2[0]} \qquad (5.15)$$

and therefore

$$C_1(x) = C_2(x) \qquad (5.16)$$

indicating that nowhere in the hairpin countercurrent system can there be a difference in the osmotic pressure between the two limbs. If this is the case, then eqn (5.10) can be written more simply

$$\Delta p = p \qquad (5.10a)$$

The solution of the differential equation derived from eqns (5.10a), (5.12a and b) and (5.13) which reduced to:

$$\frac{dV_1}{dx} = -\frac{dV_2}{dx} = -\frac{yp}{a} \qquad (5.17)$$

gives:

$$(V_1)_x = -(V_2) = V_{1[0]} - \frac{yp}{a} \cdot x \qquad (5.18)$$

In a steady state, the concentrations at a point x of the hairpin countercurrent system can be calculated from eqn (5.15)

$$C_x = C_{1[0]} \frac{V_{1[0]}}{Vx} = C_{1[0]} \frac{1}{1 - (yp/aV_{1[0]})x} \qquad (5.19)$$

whereas the highest concentration reached at the bend will be

$$C_{max} = c(L) = C_{1[0]} \frac{1}{1 - (yp/aV_{1[0]})L} \qquad (5.20)$$

From eqn (5.18) it is now possible to calculate the velocity of the flow V and to determine its value at two different points x_α and x_β.
Thus:

$$(V_1)_{x_\alpha} = (V_1)_{x_\beta} - \frac{yp}{a}(x_\alpha - x_\beta) \qquad (5.19a)$$

which when expressed in terms of concentration c or of a concentrating factor (f) becomes:

$$_\beta^\alpha f = \frac{C(x_\alpha)}{C(x_\beta)} = \frac{1}{[1 - (yp/aV_\beta)] \cdot (x_\alpha - x_\beta)} \qquad (5.21)$$

Thus from the concentration $c(x_\alpha)$ and $c(x_\beta)$ which can be estimated at two different sites x_α and x_β of the hairpin countercurrent system, it is possible to determine the magnitude of the parameter yp/aV_β. Hence it is possible to determine the concentration at any point of the system.

From the eqn (5.20), giving the maximum concentration, it will be seen that for C_{max} to be large the quantity $(yp/aV_{1[0]}).L$ must have a value close to 1. In that case $c(L)=\infty$, a case which is not likely to occur. Likewise, one could imagine a negative concentration if $(yp/aV_{1[0]}).L>1$. But this could never happen.

It is clear then that the magnitude of the longitudinal gradient established in a hairpin countercurrent system will depend on (a) the magnitude of the 'single effect' at any point, (b) the length of the loop along which the single effect is multiplied and (c) the

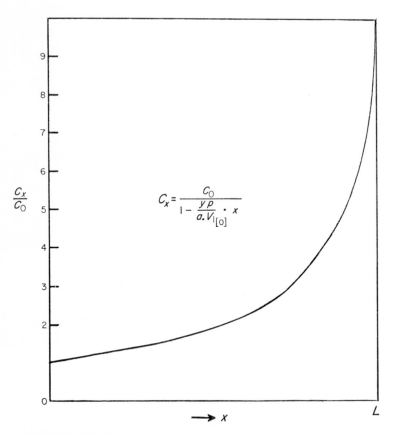

$$C_x = \frac{C_0}{1 - \frac{y\,p}{a.V_{1[0]}} \cdot x}$$

FIG. 5.5. Development of a concentration in a hairpin countercurrent mechanism. The example refers to a ten-fold increase of concentration. For explanation of symbols, see text.

volume-flow through the loop. As long as the semipermeability of the membrane separating the two limbs remains constant throughout its length water movement from one limb to another will produce an osmotic gradient which will rise not linearly but hyperbolically.

In the model used by Hargitay & Kuhn (1951), in which fluid is transiently concentrated in a countercurrent multiplier as a result of hydrostatic difference, the parameter $(yp/aV_{1[0]})L = 0.9$ and the concentration of the fluid at the point x is given as

$$c_x = \frac{c_0}{1 - (yp/aV_{1[0]}) \cdot x} \qquad (5.22)$$

where c_x = concentration of solution at point x, c_0 = concentration of entering fluid, a = cross-sectional area of the limbs, $V_{1[0]}$ = the linear velocity of inflowing fluid, y = the water permeability of membrane, and p = the hydrostatic pressure difference across the membrane.

The analysis of the hairpin countercurrent system as presented here has followed closely the more detailed mathematical treatment of the problem presented by Hargitay & Kuhn (1951). These authors showed also the mathematical consequences that would result from the withdrawal of some of the concentrated fluid either, (a) from the bend of the loop, or (b) by a third adjacent tube running parallel with the inflow current, but separated from the limb by a water-permeable membrane. Such a tube might be considered analogous to the collecting duct in the kidney.

The ideas expounded by Hargitay & Kuhn (1951), Hargitay et al. (1951) and Wirz et al. (1951) were not easily accepted by physiologists who had been nurtured on the views of Smith and his coworkers. Smith (1959) pointed out that Hargitay & Kuhn's concept was based on the presence of a hydrostatic pressure, and that without it there would not be a 'single effect'. Hargitay & Kuhn emphatically denied that hydrostatic pressure was the operative concentrating force in the kidney. In their own words, this is what they said: 'Auf alle Fälle steht, wie wir weiter unten festellen werden, fest, dass es sich dabei um *keinen* hydrostatischen sondern veraussichtlich um einen elektroosmotischen Druck handelt.' In 1959, Kuhn & Ramel presented a new mathematical treatment of a countercurrent multiplier which appeared to be more closely related to functions of the concentrating kidney. The driving force was taken to be the active transport of sodium, which would operate from the ascending to the descending limb of the loop. In this model the maximum concentrating ability was directly proportional to the driving force, and conductance, of the membrane for the actively transported ion, and inversely proportional to the volume-flow through the countercurrent multiplier. The mathematical treatment of this model is rather complicated and a detailed consideration of it is not justified as it rests on two unwarranted assumptions; first, that the two limbs of the loop of Henle are separated by a membrane impermeable to water, but responsible for the active transport of sodium; and second, that the descending limb of the system is in contact with the collecting tube through a membrane permeable to water but impermeable to sodium.

Hargitay & Kuhn's work stimulated others to produce improved theoretical models. Pinter & Shohet (1963) pointed out that, in the hypotheses of Hargitay & Kuhn (1951) and Kuhn & Ramel (1959), the presence of the collecting ducts was considered, but the role of the vasa recta had been omitted as an integral part of the system. On the other hand, Thurau, Deetjen & Gunzler (1962) derived equations for the concentration profile in the vasa recta, but did not incorporate the loops of Henle. Furthermore, though most models were successful in predicting most of the experimental results obtained from chemical analysis of the medulla of a concentrating kidney, they did not offer a satisfactory explanation for the sodium concentration found in the medulla during water diuresis. In an attempt to answer some of these criticisms, Pinter & Shohet (1963) presented a model whose central feature was that the countercurrent multiplier of the loop of Henle was restricted to the thick segment of the ascending limb. By including the vasa recta in their calculations, they sought to prove that the interstitial sodium concentration could increase in the papilla, but to achieve this they had to assume that the collecting duct contributed a constant amount of solute and/or water to the medullary interstitium along its entire length. This, however, was criticized by Stephenson (1965) who, in a complicated analysis of the differential equations describing a two-loop system of vasa recta and loop of Henle, pointed out that a system of the kind presented by Pinter & Shohet (1963) would not be able either to concentrate or dilute, as expected from a countercurrent system; i.e. it could not produce a concentration either greater or less than the maximum or minimum concentrations of the fluid entering it. According to Stephenson (1966), Kelman & Marsh produced a similar analysis of the two-loop system and reached the same conclusion.

In 1966, Stephenson extended some of the ideas he had introduced in his previous (1965) paper and gave an analysis of counterflow systems with any number of loops. Without going into the complicated mathematical treatment of the author, his conclusion was that, since all the differential equations describing the different systems used indicated that the concentrations of outflowing solutions lie between the maximum and the minimum concentrations of the entering solution, these systems could not be accepted as concentrating mechanisms. The systems analysed, however, did not include either hydrostatic pressure or pressure-flow relations and considered a single solute only. The limitation of this type of model comes from thermodynamic considerations. If there is a single inflow of a solution of salt and water of a given osmolality and if, in the countercurrent system, some combination of processes takes place by which this single inflow can be separated into two outflows each of different osmolality, this cannot be achieved without work being done. If, however, there are two or more inflowing solutions, each with different concentrations, there is no reason why they could not be coupled in an osmotic 'engine' which could perform useful work. This work could then be used to concentrate another part of the inflow and eventually produce an outflow with a higher concentration than that of the inflow. This, however, cannot be done without some process in the system able to transport the solute from a region of lower to one of higher concentration or to move the solvent from a region of higher to one of lower solute concentration. In either case, this requires the performance of work at the site of transport. It so happens that none of the systems presented have made any provision for performing work of concentration. The processes going on in them consist entirely of diffusion of sodium along a concentration gradient, passive transfer of sodium across a membrane, or transport with no pressure differential.

So far the discussion has evolved in terms of a theoretical analysis of the multiplication of a 'single effect' which does not appear to be relevant to the physiology of the kidney. From the previous chapter it would seem that the mechanism of concentration in the kidney depends primarily on the existence of a process which raises the osmolar concentration of tissue fluid and constituent structures of the innermost part of the medulla. This primary process of osmotic concentration in the papilla has been attributed to the active reabsorption of sodium chloride in a region of the nephron before the distal tubule, some of the salt remaining in the tissue fluid and raising its concentration. That the concentration is graded, with its maximum towards the papilla, is consistent with its being produced by a countercurrent mechanism in which the single effect would be initiated by the active transport of sodium.

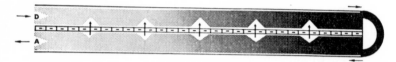

FIG. 5.6. Diagram illustrating the action of the hairpin countercurrent system, in producing a great increase in concentration at tip of the hairpin. A: ascending loop of Henle, D: descending loop of Henle. The stippling indicates the corresponding increase in concentration of the fluid towards the tip of the loop. ↑ represents reabsorption of Na from the ascending into the descending loops.

Take a tube divided along its middle by a septum which, instead of being semipermeable as in the model proposed by Hargitay & Kuhn (1951), has the property of actively transporting sodium chloride from the lower side A (Fig. 5.6) to the upper side D. If a solution of sodium chloride enters the tube at D, owing to the property of the salt-transporting septum, the concentration of the solution in channel D will steadily rise, while that in the compartment A will steadily fall. Since the two channels A and D of the tube are joined together at one end by a U-tube, the concentration of the solution entering channel A will be the same as that leaving channel D. Thus, the solution at the tip of the hairpin will be at a much higher concentration than that of the solution either entering or leaving the channels. This higher concentration will be the result of a multiplication of a single effect as would be created by each single element of the septum if there were no countercurrent, and it might increase indefinitely with increase in the length of the whole system as in the theoretical models of Hargitay & Kuhn (1951) and Kuhn & Ramel (1959).

Applying this idea to the kidney of mammals, the hairpin system will be identified with the loop of Henle, the ascending loop being channel A of Fig. 5.6, the cells of its wall acting as the salt transporting system. Since in the kidney the descending and the ascending limbs are not two separate channels of a single tube, but are separated by interstitial tissue and blood vessels, the transfer of sodium chloride from the ascending limb will not be directly into the descending limb, but into the interstitial fluid from which it is supposed to diffuse passively through the thin walls of the descending limb. The loop of Henle acting as a hairpin countercurrent system will maintain a gradient of concentration in the interstitial fluid, which will increase from the region of both the proximal and the distal convoluted tubules to the tip of the loop deep in the papilla.

Since in the hairpin countercurrent system, as represented either by Fig. 5.6 or by the loops of Henle in the kidney (Fig. 5.7), the solution leaving it has the same concentration as that entering it, the system cannot by itself yield a concentrated urine. To achieve this, it is necessary to postulate that the walls of the collecting ducts are permeable to water but not to any of the substances in solution. If this is so, the solution entering the collecting ducts will have the same concentration as that of the solution leaving the distal tubules, but as it flows through the collecting ducts, in the direction of the papilla, it will lose water by osmosis into the hairpin system and thus become more concentrated and osmotic work will be performed. Since it would be useless to have water transferred into the countercurrent system, it must be carried away by the blood, as otherwise the whole process of concentration would soon come to an end. As vasa recta are similar to all other lower pressure capillaries, they will be able to draw fluid into the blood from the tissue spaces and so remove the excess water.

This short account of the formation of concentrated urine based on the active reabsorptive process of sodium is in complete agreement with the theory of a hairpin countercurrent multiplication system, which Hargitay & Kuhn (1951) presented initially as 'an exercise in physiological speculation'. It may not have answered all the questions or solved all the problems; it remains, however,

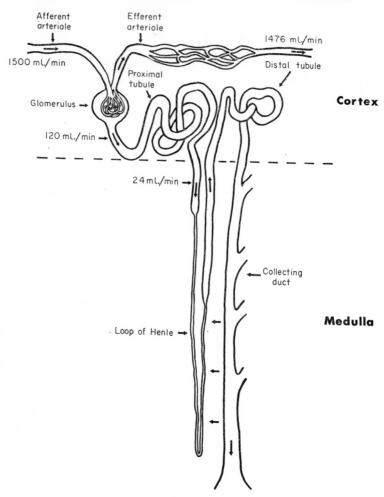

Fig. 5.7. Representation of a nephron and its relation to the cortex and medulla in the kidney. The two limbs of the loop of Henle form a hairpin countercurrent system. The numerals represent the approximate volume of fluid passing through the different parts of the nephron.

an up-to-date mathematical and physical analysis of what appears to happen in the kidneys of mammals. It is correct (Berliner *et al.*, 1958) that it may contain an apparent 'internal contradiction', namely that to be effective the loop of Henle must be permeable to water, though in order for a high osmotic concentration to exist within the loop, the latter must be impermeable to water. But in spite of this, most of the essential features of the countercurrent multiplier theory have been subsequently confirmed by experiments.

6

COUNTERCURRENT SYSTEM AND LOOP OF HENLE

IT is tempting to postulate that the thin segment of the loop of Henle plays a major role in the make-up of the osmotic profile in the inner medulla. It raises, however, several problems. If there is a process of countercurrent multiplication in the thin loop, this will require that sodium is actively transported through the water-impermeable membrane of the thin ascending limb. Since the descending limb is permeable to water a change of permeability of the membrane to water must occur at the bend of the loop. This has been criticized on two grounds: first, histologically there is little difference between the thin descending and ascending limbs; second, there is no evidence to suggest that the cells of the ascending limb can provide the energy necessary for the active transport of this ion (Smith, 1959). In support of the suggestion, however, is the observation that in the hamster and the rat the lumen of the thin descending limb widens just before the bend of the loop (Gottschalk, 1964).

The best evidence for the existence of a hairpin countercurrent system in the loop of Henle comes from micropuncture studies. Most of them, however, have been performed on the golden hamster only. Even in the hands of skilled workers such as Gottschalk these experiments are technically difficult and liable to errors. Furthermore, they can provide only limited information, since it is only a short portion of the papilla that is accessible. The precise determination of the chemical composition of the fluid collected in the several parts of the papilla is fraught with difficulties. Finally, the interpretation of the results is rendered difficult owing to the fall in concentrating ability of the kidney that generally occurs during the time required for collection. Nevertheless, in spite of it all, micropuncture techniques have been uniquely helpful in establishing the physiological role of the loop of Henle.

The difficulty in interpreting the results can be illustrated by the following examples. According to Gottschalk (1964) about 66% of sodium salt and 19% of urea account for the total osmolality of the fluid collected from the bend of the loop of Henle. Whether these percentages can be extrapolated to conditions of maximum urine concentration is still unknown. During antidiuresis, urine collected from sites in the collecting ducts at the same level as the bend in the papilla has the same osmolality as the fluid sampled from the loop but differs in its chemical composition: its concentration of urea is greater while the concentration of sodium is lower. The concentrations of urea and chloride in blood from the vasa recta have been found to be intermediate between those in the fluid of the loop of Henle and those in the collecting ducts, and since the osmolality of the fluids in collecting ducts, in the vasa recta and at the bend of the loop is the same, one might expect that the concentration of sodium in blood could be lower than in the fluid from the loop (Gottschalk, 1964). Such conclusions, however, do not always agree with results of direct estimations of sodium chloride in the blood from the vasa recta (Ullrich, Pehling & Espinar-Lafuente (1961).

This is another example. Thurau, Wilde, Henne, Schnermann & Prchal (1963), using a timed photomicrographical method to follow the passage of a dye injected into the lumen of the loop, estimated the flow through the thin descending and thin ascending limbs during antidiuresis and during induced osmotic diuresis in the hamster. The rate of flow in the thin descending limb during antidiuresis was estimated at 31.4×10^{-9} ml./sec, while that of the thin ascending limb was 37.7×10^{-9} ml./sec. During osmotic diuresis, the rate of flow in the thin descending limb was estimated at 28×10^{-9} ml./sec, and in the thin ascending limb at 29.1×10^{-9} ml./sec. If this is so why is it that the rate of flow in the thin ascending limb is appreciably lower during osmotic diuresis than during antidiuresis? As a reduction of filtration rate is more likely to occur during antidiuresis than during an osmotic diuresis, the reverse would be expected. Second, why is the rate of flow in the thin ascending limb so much greater than in the corresponding descending limb, during antidiuresis? Thurau et al. (1963) suggested that this could be explained if it were assumed that the fluid in the loop had a slightly higher osmolality than that of the interstitial fluid, a situation which one would expect in a countercurrent diffusion exchanger and which would produce an influx of water and hence an increase of flow. This, however, is conjectural since no determination of the osmolality of interstitial fluid was made.

Gertz (1963) injected into the lumen of a renal tubule a column of oil which he split by subsequent injection of a droplet of an aqueous solution. The rate of reabsorption of the aqueous drop was calculated from serial observations of changes in its length. From the time-course of reabsorption of various solutions injected Gertz (1963) deduced important characteristics for the permeability and the transport through the epithelium of the proximal and distal tubules. This technique, initially devised for the study of convoluted tubules, was subsequently adapted for the investigation of the functions of the loop of Henle by at least two groups of research workers; unfortunately their results were different and sometimes conflicting. According to Marsh & Solomon (1965), who used Gertz's technique for the loop of Henle in hamsters undergoing osmotic diuresis, neither the descending nor the ascending limb reabsorbed a solution of sodium chloride. Thus according to these authors there is no active transport by either limb, descending or ascending. Gottschalk (1964), on the other hand, also using Gertz's technique but in non-diuretic hamsters, found evidence of reabsorption of injected droplets of isotonic, hypotonic or hypertonic solutions of sodium chloride in the thin descending limb of the loop of Henle, but not in the thin ascending limb. In the ascending limb, the injected droplets underwent changes in their chemical composition: whether the droplets were of distilled water or of sodium chloride solutions, either isotonic, hypotonic or hypertonic, when they were reaspirated, their osmolality was always similar to that of the fluid from the collecting ducts. From these observations Gottschalk (1964) concluded that while osmotic equilibration involving only solute movement occurred in the thin ascending limb, in the thin descending limb there was movement of both water and solute, a clear indication of a difference in the functional properties of the two limbs.

The fact that droplets containing solutes of different concentrations are reabsorbed when injected in the lumen of the thin descending limb, raises the question whether this is due to a mechanism of bulk filtration or to active transport of sodium.

Though the possibility of bulk filtration cannot be dismissed, the fact that reabsorption of droplets occurred in limbs which had been decompressed through puncture holes near the column of oil makes it improbable. Furthermore, though active sodium reabsorption could not be demonstrated, it is nevertheless the most likely mechanism since it is consistent with the existence of a difference of the transtubular electrical potential across the limb. During free-flow, the average potential difference in the descending and ascending limbs has been estimated at -3 and -11 mV, respectively (Windhager, 1965).

Since any potential difference measured was shown to arise locally, and was not transmitted from other parts of the nephron, electrophysiological studies of the renal papilla of hamsters have contributed substantially to the understanding of the functions of both limbs of the loop of Henle. When the loop was perfused with an hypertonic solution of 1.8% sodium chloride containing a metabolic inhibitor such as potassium cyanide or iodoacetic acid, the potential difference in the descending limb changed from -3 to $+1$ mV and that in the ascending limb from -11 to $+8.9$ mV, but they returned to their respective normal values when the inhibitors were withdrawn. These results were interpreted by Windhager (1965) as indicating the existence of active transport of both sodium and chloride across the epithelium of the thin ascending limb.

From the experiments by Gottschalk (1964) and Windhager (1965), the following picture seems to emerge: the thin ascending limb is impermeable to water, but not to sodium or chloride, while the thin descending limb is permeable to water. This alone, however, is not enough to prove that the loop of Henle functions as a countercurrent system, unless it can be shown that the fluid in the descending limb is iso-osmotic, while that in the ascending limb is slightly hypo-osmotic, with the interstitial fluid.

The vasa recta were at first considered as a system of straight tubular structures. They differ, however, from this as they do not form loops but are connected together through capillary plexuses (Moffat & Fourman, 1963). It is thought, without much experimental evidence, that the vasa recta operate passively as a countercurrent diffusion exchanger, allowing the passage of ions along their electrochemical gradients. If this is so they cannot contribute to the establishment of osmotic gradients, though their role in minimizing salt loss should not be overlooked.

Thurau *et al.* (1963) measured a fall of blood pressure of 6·5 mm/Hg per mm length of the descending vasa in the exposed papilla in the hamster. From this they estimated that the fall in pressure along the entire descending vasa recta would be of the order of 40 mm Hg or more. This presumed that a high pressure would be in keeping with the relatively large diameter of the efferent arterioles of the juxta-medullary glomeruli. These findings have been used to support the hypothesis that the vasa recta might function as a countercurrent multiplier system activated by a gradient of hydrostatic pressure. Quite apart from the fact that this explanation was explicitly discarded by Hargitay & Kuhn (1951), one would have to assume that the endothelium of these capillaries was more permeable to water than to electrolytes for this mechanism to be functional. Furthermore, the anatomical arrangement of these capillaries would have to be such as to permit the direct passage of water from the ascending into the descending limbs and to prevent at the same time the access of water into other areas of the medulla. For these reasons, Gottschalk (1964) considered that the existence of a 'countercurrent multiplication in the vasa recta as a possible mechanism for increasing sodium and osmotic concentration in the inner zone . . . is unlikely'.

There are, however, other reasons for accepting that a countercurrent mechanism is at work in the kidney. Morel, Guinnebault & Amiel (1960) injected hamsters intravenously with a solution of radioactive sodium in tritiated water and estimated the sodium and the water content in different regions of the kidney. Similar experiments were performed in rabbits (Morel & Guinnebault, 1961). In both species it could be shown that in the cortex, tritiated water was equilibrated with plasma water almost at once, whereas in the medulla and even more so in the papilla, the process of equilibration took a much longer time – up to 10 min in the hamster and up to 60 min in the rabbit. Radioactive sodium, on the other hand, established equilibrium with the plasma water almost at once, whether in the cortex, the medulla or the papilla.

Lassen & Longley (1961) worked on the assumption that 'where a gradient for any diffusible material exists between its two ends, a countercurrent exchanger acts as a barrier to the net transport of that material along its long axis'. In other words, the more diffusible the material, the more effective the barrier. Thus in a passive system, concentrations of sodium, chloride and urea would be conserved more effectively than concentrations of larger molecules, but less effectively than gases. To demonstrate this, they performed two different types of experiments: in the first, non-anaesthetized rats were made to breathe radioactive krypton, ^{85}Kr, in a concentration of 50 μc/ml. air. At varying times, animals were dropped into liquid nitrogen, and radioautographs were prepared by placing X-ray films in contact with still frozen sections of the body and concentrations of ^{85}Kr estimated by densitometry. In all experiments, in less than 1 minute after inhalation of the gas, the concentration of radioactive krypton in the renal cortex was similar to that of the blood, suggesting that the cortex was saturated with the inert gas, but it took up to 90 minutes for radioautographs of the kidney to show an average density of the papilla equal to 93% of that of the cortex. These results confirmed those of Morel et al. (1960) with radioactive sodium.

In the other series of experiments, two substances of widely different diffusion characteristics were infused into kidneys in situ. The substances added to the perfusate were either radioactive sodium ^{24}Na and ^{131}I iodinated serum albumin or ^{131}I antipyrine and ^{198}Au colloidal gold. With ^{131}I iodinated serum albumin, however, the incorporation of albumin in the papilla was much faster than in the cortex. Thus the incorporation of a large molecule in the papilla was faster than with a highly diffusible gas. When ^{131}I iodinated serum albumin and ^{24}Na were infused together, the cortex incorporated them about 6 times as rapidly as did the papilla. The use of ^{131}I antipyrine and ^{198}Au yielded similar results. This again confirmed the experiments by Morel et al. (1960) using tritiated water and radioactive sodium. Lassen & Longley (1961) concluded from these experiments that the 'countercurrent action of the renal medullary vasculature, apparently passive, is demonstrated by its differential exclusion of materials from the papilla of the kidney in order of diffusibility'.

Other evidence of the existence of a countercurrent system in the kidney is provided by the exchange of oxygen between the two limbs of the loops. According to Auckland & Krog (1960a, b) the partial pressure of oxygen in the kidney decreases steadily from the cortex down to the papilla. Two years earlier, Rennie, Reeves & Pappenheimer (1958) had noticed that oxygen of the urine in the pelvis had a partial pressure markedly lower than that in the efferent venous blood from the kidney. Though the interpretation given by Rennie et al. (1958) of this observation may not have been the correct one, it can be explained by an equilibration of the partial pressure of oxygen between the urine in the collecting ducts and the low partial pressure of oxygen in the medulla and the papilla.

A mechanism of countercurrent exchange has also been invoked for other gases than oxygen, such as krypton (Longley, Lassen & Lilienfeld, 1958) and CO_2. When urine is alkaline, the partial pressure of CO_2 in the urine is markedly in excess of that in the blood of the renal artery or renal vein (Ochwadt & Pitts, 1956); when, however, the urine is acid, the partial pressure of CO_2 in urine is very low (Brodsky, Miley, Kaim & Shah, 1958). Ullrich (1959) suggested that this too could be explained by the existence of a countercurrent exchange mechanism. It is well known that acidification of the urine proceeds along the collecting ducts as a cationic exchange between the reabsorption of Na ions and the secretion of hydrogen ions (Ullrich & Eigler, 1958; Gottschalk, Lassiter & Mylle, 1960). Thus, when a strongly acid urine is elaborated, the high amount of CO_2, required to produce the carbonic acid and hence by hydrolysis the hydrogen ions, may quite well exceed the amount of CO_2 produced by cellular metabolism, which would lead to the establishment of a negative gradient of the concentration of CO_2 in the tissue; inversely, when the urine is very alkaline, the amount of CO_2 utilized would be much smaller than that produced in the renal medulla, and hence the establishment of a positive gradient of concentration. In this way the hypothesis of gas exchange by countercurrent in the inner medulla would account for the observation, otherwise inexplicable, of the difference between the partial pressures of O_2 and CO_2 in urine and blood.

This interpretation is supported by the findings of Kramer (1962) who, from estimations of O_2 consumption and of blood flow in the medulla, showed that there is an A–V oxygen difference between the in- and the out-flowing blood of the vasa recta amounting to 1–2 vol. %, whereas the difference of O_2 uptake between artery and papilla ($A_{O_2} - P_{O_2}$) amounts to 14 vol. % O_2. These results would agree with the views that oxygen is being 'short-circuited' in the outer zone of the medulla. Kramer, Deetjen & Brechtelsbauer (1961) also showed that any change of oxygen concentration in the in-flowing blood through the vasa recta leads to a change of the steady state of the gradient of concentration, the duration of the change depending on the rate of flow of the blood. Thus, during antidiuresis a new state for O_2 gradient would be achieved in some six minutes, while during osmotic diuresis this time is considerably shortened.

The very low concentration of oxygen observed in the renal medulla, of course, raises the question of aerobic metabolism of the cells. Forty years ago, Gyorgy, Keller & Brehme (1928) found that tissue slices from the renal medulla, even when incubated in the presence of oxygen, are the site of anaerobic glycolysis, leading to the formation of lactic acid. This was confirmed by Dickens & Weil-Malherbe (1936), but challenged by Ruiz-Guinazu, Pehling, Rumrich & Ullrich (1961) and by Ullrich (1962). Plasma was obtained from blood collected by micropuncture from vasa recta at the tip of the papilla of hamsters and analysed for its content of glucose and lactic acid. The results showed that the concentration of lactic acid was significantly higher ($+21$ mg %) and that of glucose considerably lower (-57 mg %) than in the arterial blood plasma. On the assumption that these compounds diffuse across a countercurrent system, Ullrich (1962) calculated that 25% of the glucose utilized would appear as lactic acid. If 75% of the glucose were oxidized, *in vivo*, the ratio Q_{O_2}/Q_{CO_2} would be 9, whereas *in vitro* experiments this ratio is of the order of 0·5. Thus, it would appear that at least in the renal papilla of the hamster *in vivo* the aerobic metabolism prevails. This, however, does not agree very well with the results of Weinstein & Klose (1969) in the rat.

Though the essential features of a countercurrent multiplier system appear to exist in the renal medulla evidence that the loops of Henle and/or the vasa recta are capable of performing osmotic work was still lacking. In 1967, Jamison, Bennett & Berliner succeeded in demonstrating that a difference in the osmolality between the two limbs of the loop existed, the fluid in the ascending limb having an osmotic pressure significantly lower than that in the descending limb. This was shown in adult male rats. During a first operation, using a modification of the technique devised by Sakai, Jamison & Berliner (1965) a part of the cortex was removed and the renal medulla exposed. In a second operation, the anaesthetized rat was infused intravenously with a 0·9% sodium chloride solution containing 4 mμ vasopressin/ml. An area of the exposed papilla

D

was selected in which at least two limbs of the loops of Henle passed close together. The external diameter of the pipettes used for puncture of the limbs was between 5 and 7 μ at the tip; that of the pipettes used for puncturing the blood vessels between 8 and 11 μ. To ascertain the direction of the flow in the limbs, one was punctured and a small drop of oil injected into the lumen. If the punctured tubule was an ascending limb, the fluid was collected slowly enough to allow the droplet of oil to flow away. If, on the other hand, the tubule punctured was a descending limb, the rate of entry of fluid into the pipette was kept as low as possible. After the first puncture, the pipette was removed, its tip sealed, the site of puncture noted and its location measured with a micrometer. The second loop was then punctured at the same level and as close as possible to the first puncture site. The time between the onset of the first and the completion of the second collections averaged 10 minutes. In some experiments, a collecting duct was punctured after the loops, but in animals where the vasa recta were punctured, this was done always at the end of the experiment since the bleeding prevented further observations from being made. Samples of less than 1 nl. were used for the estimation of osmolality using the Ramsay and Brown (1955) microcryoscopic technique. Plasma of blood from the vasa recta was separated from the red cells by gravity and transferred to a second pipette for cryoscopic estimations. After determination of the freezing point, samples were analysed for their sodium and potassium content, using the dual-channel helium-glow ultramicrophotometer of Vurek and Bowman (1965). In a third series of experiments, 2–4 days after the operation, rats were anaesthetized again, their ureters cannulated and the glomerular filtration rate estimated by means of inulin clearance.

Three groups of comparison were made: the concentration of the fluid collected close to the hairpin bend was compared with that from an adjacent descending limb taken at the same level; fluids from two adjacent descending limbs were compared and finally fluid from an ascending limb was compared with that from an adjacent descending limb. In another series of experiments, fluid from descending limbs was compared with the plasma from descending vasa recta, and lastly the fluid from the descending limb and hairpin bend of the loop of Henle was compared with the plasma from ascending vasa recta. The results showed that

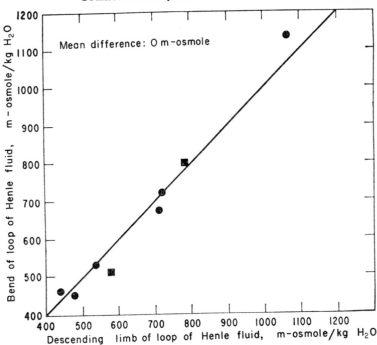

FIG. 6.1. Comparison of osmolalities of fluid from descending limbs and adjacent hairpin turns of the loop of Henle. Solid line indicates identity. ●, ascending limb of bend; ■, descending limb of bend (from Jamison, Bennett & Berliner, 1967).

there was no difference between the osmolality of the fluids collected at the bend of the loop and in the descending limb (Fig. 6.1), and that there was no significant difference between the osmolality of fluids collected from two descending limbs (Fig. 6.2). When, however, the fluids from the descending and ascending limb were compared (Fig. 6.3), the fluid in the ascending limb was found to have a significantly lower osmolality than that in the descending limb, the mean difference being -117 m-osmole/kg H_2O, $P<0.001$. Furthermore, fluid from the descending limb had a significantly higher osmolality than the plasma of the vasa recta (mean difference: $+64$ m-osmole/kg H_2O, $P<0.001$). In contrast, fluid from the ascending limb and plasma from the descending vasa recta had the same osmolality, which suggests a time lag in the establishment of osmotic equilibrium between the blood of the

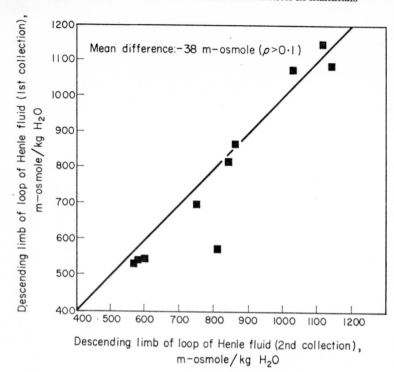

FIG. 6.2. Comparison of osmolalities of fluid from adjacent descending limbs of the loop of Henle (from Jamison *et al.* 1967).

vasa recta and their surroundings. Finally (Fig. 6.6), they found no appreciable difference between the osmolality of the fluid from either the descending limb or the hairpin bend of the loop of Henle and of the plasma from the ascending vasa recta. In 19 pairs of collections from the ascending and descending limbs, a total osmolality of 772·9 and 939·2 m-osmole/kg H_2O was found respectively, with corresponding values for sodium of 257·2 and 329·3 m-equiv/l. It was calculated that the osmolality in the ascending and descending limbs due to the concentration of NaCl was 473·2 and 605·8 m-osmole/kg H_2O respectively. As for the potassium, similar amounts of 19·9 and 20·9 m-equiv/l. were found in both limbs.

The results of this investigation, which is the most complete and thorough so far, support conclusively the hypothesis that the descending thin limb acts as a countercurrent multiplier and that

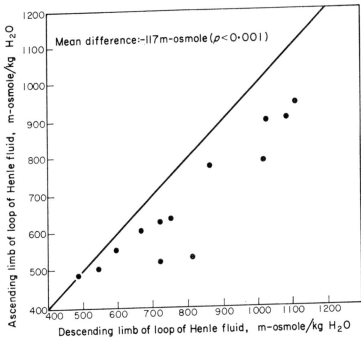

FIG. 6.3. Comparison of osmolalities of fluid from ascending limbs and adjacent descending limbs of the loop of Henle (from Jamison *et al.*, 1967).

the 'single effect' is the dilution of the fluid in the thin ascending limb by active transport of sodium, or sodium chloride. It will be remembered that in 1964 Gottschalk hesitated to draw any conclusions as to the functional differences between ascending and descending limbs. It would appear, however, that after a recent analysis of a large number of samples from the thin limbs of the hamster, he too found that the fluid of the ascending limb had a lower osmolality than that collected from the descending limb (see footnote in Jamison *et al.*, 1967). It can therefore be accepted that there is a change of permeability of the cells of the loop and that soon after the hairpin bend, the thin ascending limb becomes relatively impermeable to water, so that removal of the solutes, mostly if not entirely NaCl, renders the fluid hypo-osmotic to the surrounding tissue.

It has been argued that the loops of Henle lack cytological specialization usually associated with active transport processes.

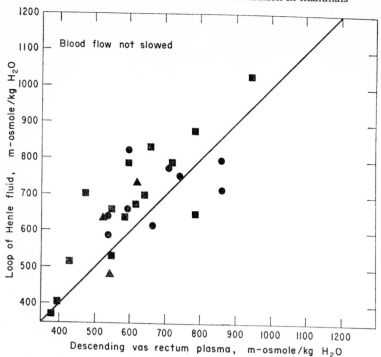

Fig. 6.4. Comparison of osmolalities of fluid from loops of Henle and plasma from adjacent descending vasa recta in which the flow of blood did not appear to be slowed (from Jamison *et al.*, 1967.) Henle's loop: ■, descending limb mean difference $+74$ $(p<0\cdot01)$; ●, ascending limb mean difference $+35$ $(p>0\cdot3)$; ▲, bend mean difference $+65$. Total $=27$.

Since all living cells so far investigated have the property of expelling sodium ions by means of a 'pump' (Bayliss, 1966), one could accept that in all likelihood the cells of the loops are not different in this respect from any other living cells. One can, however, go further: a characteristic of all epithelial cells transporting actively is the presence at the inner surface of tight intercellular junctions, called terminal bars, which have been described for the thin loop of Henle by Rhodin (1958); and by Farquhar & Palade (1963). The energy needed for the working of the pump comes usually from the combination with oxygen of the sugar glucose. The paucity of mitochondria and other organelles (Wachstein & Bradshaw, 1965), however, may suggest that the cells lining the

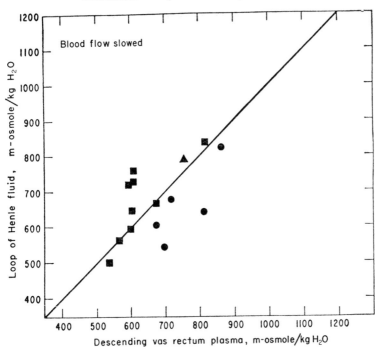

FIG. 6.5. Comparison of osmolalities of fluid from loops of Henle and plasma from adjacent descending vasa recta in which the blood flow was slowed (from Jamison *et al.*, 1967). Henle's loop: ■, descending limb mean difference $+45$ ($p \sim 0.1$); ●, ascending limb mean difference -95 ($p < 0.025$); ▲, bend. Total $= 15$.

thin loops of Henle derive some of their energy from sources other than the usual oxidative process. This would agree with the low oxygen tension (Kramer, *et al.*, 1960) and the high concentration of lactate found in the renal medulla (Ruiz-Guinazu *et al.*, 1961; Scaglione, Dell & Winters, 1965).

Recently Lapp & Nolte (1962) and Oswaldo & Latta (1966) have presented electron microscopic studies from which there would appear to be a difference between the structure of the descending and that of the ascending limbs. In contrast to the ascending limb, the descending limb has microvilli and infoldings of the basal membrane, whereas the basal membrane of the ascending limb is stratified (Lapp & Nolte, 1962). The cellular modifications which appear to be specific to each thin limb are striking near the end of

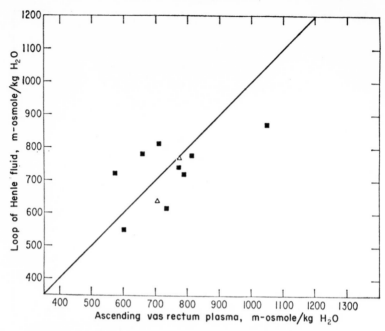

FIG. 6.6. Comparison of osmolalities of fluid from loops of Henle and plasma from adjacent ascending vasa recta (from Jamison *et al.*, 1967). Henle's loop: ■, descending limb; Δ, bend. Mean difference of both from ascending vas rectum −19 ($p > 0.5$).

the thin segment but do not appear to exist at the bend of the loop. These observations go a long way towards providing an anatomical support for the physiological findings of Berliner and his associates (Jamison *et al.*, 1967). Whereas the fluid in the bend of the loop is in osmotic equilibrium with the fluid in an adjacent descending thin limb at about 1 mm above the bend, changes of the basal membrane of the thin ascending limb have been observed which would be compatible with a change of permeability to water.

Electron-microscopic differences have also been described for the descending and the ascending vasa recta (Longley, Banfield & Brindley, 1959; Brewer, 1965) and may well account for the time lag observed in the osmotic equilibrium between the descending vasa recta and adjacent loops of Henle. The magnitude of the difference between the osmotic pressure (average 75 m-osmoles) is difficult to understand as ordinary capillary membranes have in general a high coefficient of filtration (Pappenheimer, 1953; Bayliss, 1960). Since, however, the difference between the osmolality of the descending vasa recta and the fluid in the thin descending limb disappears when the flow through the vasa recta is slowed down (Figs. 6.4 and 6.5), it is not unreasonable to assume, as suggested by Berliner, that the osmolality of the entering blood may be influenced by the linear rate of flow in vessels passing through a region of continuously increasing osmolality. Whatever the explanation, it must be realized that if no difference in the osmolality of the descending vasa recta and the fluid in the adjacent descending limb existed, the vasa recta could not function as passive countercurrent exchangers. In this respect it is of some interest to record that, according to Lever (1965), the process of multiplication occurs in the vasa recta and not in the loops of Henle. This is based on the assumption that the single effect is the result of an ultrafiltration initiated by the hydrostatic pressure in the descending vasa recta. If this were correct, however, one would expect that the osmotic pressure in the descending vasa recta would be higher than in the descending thin limb, a fact that has not been substantiated. Furthermore, as pointed out by Berliner (Jamison et al., 1967) the highest hydrostatic pressure in descending vasa recta has been estimated to be of the order of 50 mm Hg, which could account at most for an osmolality difference of 3 m-osmoles. This would be the maximum single effect which would have to be multiplied up to 1000 times, as in some rodents, and against which longitudinal diffusion within the blood stream would operate. But even if this were possible, the difference of 3 m-osmoles resulting from an hydrostatic pressure of 50 mm Hg would necessitate the complete impermeability of the capillary vessels to sodium chloride!

On the present evidence then, the single effect without which no multiplication can occur (Hargitay & Kuhn, 1951) is initiated by the dilution of the fluid in the thin ascending limb, which is multiplied by countercurrent flow within the loop of Henle to establish the osmotic gradient in the inner medulla. A similar process in the thick portion of the ascending limb would account for the osmotic gradient in the outer medulla. The role of the vasa recta would be that of a countercurrent exchange system whose function would be to preserve the established gradient.

7

EFFECTS OF VASOPRESSIN ON THE PERMEABILITY OF MEMBRANES

WITH the publication of Berliner's results (Jamison *et al.*, 1967) which established the existence of a difference in osmolality between the fluid in the descending and ascending limbs, it is now possible to assess the evolutionary role of the loops of Henle. Anatomically, the only difference between the kidney of amphibians and that of mammals is the presence in the latter of the thin segment of the loop. Since it would appear that active sodium reabsorption operates all along the renal tubule this may be accepted as a common feature of the whole nephron. The differences between the nephron of the anuran and of the mammal would therefore be narrowed down to differences in permeability characteristics of cell membranes to water. Thus in mammals the proximal convoluted tubule and the thin descending limb could be considered as functionally analogous, and so could the distal tubule and the thin ascending limb. The proximal tubule and the thin descending limb have the property of actively reabsorbing sodium and of being permeable to water, whereas in the ascending thin limb and the distal tubule, active sodium transport operates but the cells are less permeable to water. The development of the thin segment can, therefore, be visualized as an anatomical link between the two functionally different segments forming two limbs of a hairpin loop which ultimately allows multiplication by countercurrent flow.

Leaving aside the mechanism of urine concentration resulting from a reduction of glomerular filtration and from a decrease of tubular flow rates (Del Greco & De Wardener, 1956; Berliner & Davidson, 1957; Dicker, 1957), the production of hyperosmotic urine is achieved and controlled by the antidiuretic hormone. According to Smith (1956), the concentrating operation consists of a 'continuing constant reabsorbtive operation which removes an approximately constant quantity of solute-free water ($T_m^c{}_{H_2O}$) from the antecedent iso-osmotic tubular urine so long as the volume of the latter exceeds $T_m^c{}_{H_2O}$'. According to Smith (1947) this is produced by the antidiuretic hormone acting somewhere between the thin ascending loop of Henle and the distal convoluted tubule.

Results from micropuncture studies have shown that during the action of the antidiuretic hormone on the kidney of the rat, the fluid in the early part of the distal tubule is hypotonic to its surrounding milieu, but becomes iso-osmotic with it from the middle of the segment onwards (Wirz, 1956). This suggests that the antidiuretic hormone affects the permeability to water of the part of the distal tubule nearest to the collecting duct. Since, however, the fluid entering the latter is not hypertonic, the ultimate process of concentration must occur in the collecting duct and it would appear that this is achieved by allowing the osmotic pressure of the urine, as it runs down the collecting tube, to equilibrate with the osmotic pressure existing in the renal medulla.

The question then is how does the antidiuretic hormone increase the permeability to water of the collecting ducts? In view of the anatomical and functional complications of the mammalian kidney, important advances in our knowledge have been derived from experiments on the toad bladder or on the frog skin, which in the anurans have the functions assigned to the more distal portions of the nephrons in the mammal.

In the hydrated toad, the thin bilobed bladder may contain urine with a concentration of solutes as low as 50 m-osmole/kg water, thus a urine almost as dilute as that excreted by man during the peak of a water diuresis. Such dilute urine may remain in the bladder for hours without apparent decrease in volume or increase in solute concentration (Hays & Leaf, 1962).

Absence of transfer of water does not mean, however, that there is no diffusion of water. To measure the diffusion permeability, labelled water, deuterated and tritiated, is added to the medium bathing one surface of an isolated toad's bladder and its rate of appearance is estimated in the medium bathing the opposite side. To prevent the effects of solvent drag, the experiment must be done in the absence of net transfer of water. The individual labelled molecule of water will penetrate the bladder by diffusion, a process of isotopic exchange in which the driving force represented by the gradient of chemical potential of the isotope is equal to the entropy of mixing multiplied by the absolute temperature. As the 'isotopic' water molecule enters the epithelial barrier it will be subject to frictional forces between water and water and between water and membrane. The molecule will jump at random from one position to another in response to thermal agitation; it will be at one moment associated with one cluster of water molecules and at the next be part of another. Since there is no net transfer of water across the membrane, there will be no direction for the clusters to move and the progress of the labelled molecule will depend on its friction with either neighbouring water or membrane molecules. From the self-diffusion coefficient D^0, of water in water, a molecular radius of the diffusing 'species' has been calculated, using the Einstein–Stokes equation:

$$D^0 = kT/6\pi\eta r$$

where k is the Boltzmann's constant, T the absolute temperature, η the viscosity of water and r the radius of the diffusing molecule. Measurements made over a considerable range of temperatures have shown that r remains constant; its value is of approximately 1 Å, which is not very different from the calculated molecular radius of water 1·3 Å obtained from X-ray crystallography studies.

Transfer of water across a barrier in response to a gradient of hydrostatic or osmotic pressure water will depend on the movement of individual water molecules only when the dimensions of the channels through which water moves approximate the dimensions of individual molecules of water. Through all pores of larger dimensions the associated nature of water will then result in the movement of clusters of water molecules which will reduce the friction per molecule and allow larger amounts of water to be transferred for a given difference in pressure than could occur by diffusion alone. Thus while a mean pore radius of the order of 1 Å will account for diffusion, for net transfer of water it will be some 8 Å (Pappenheimer, Renkin & Borrero, 1951; Koefoed-Johnson & Ussing, 1953; Solomon, 1960; Robbins & Mauro, 1960), while under the action of vasopressin the mean pore radius would have to be of the order of 40 Å (Leaf, 1965). According to the 'pore hypothesis' water movement across a membrane (bladder or collecting tubule) occurs essentially by bulk flow through aqueous pores, rather than by diffusion, vasopressin acting by increasing the radius of individual pores. Since diffusion depends upon the area (i.e. pore radius squared) available for penetration, and since flow, according to Poiseuille's equation, varies with the fourth power of the pore radius, a small increase in pore radius will affect diffusion only by:

$$\Delta D_w = (r + \Delta r)^2 - r^2$$

whereas laminar or bulk flow will be increased by:

$$\Delta F_w = (r + \Delta r)^4 - r^4$$

Where D_w is rate of diffusional movement of water and F_w is rate of bulk flow of water Koefoed-Johnsen & Ussing (1953) suggested that the action of the antidiuretic hormone on the membrane consists mainly in altering it from one with many small pores to one with fewer but larger pores. Results of experiments on living toads bathed in solutions of different salt concentrations, in the presence and the absence of vasopressin, agree with these views (Dicker & Elliott, 1967).

Neurohypophysial hormones affect also the permeability of the isolated toad bladder to urea and acetamide, but not to thiourea. The mode of penetration by urea and similar small molecules is passive. As with water, they penetrate the bladder at equal rates in both directions, and although, in the presence of vasopressin, the coefficient of permeability for urea is increased ten-fold, the values in the two directions remain similar. An interesting experiment is that reported by Leaf and Hays (1962) in which they measured a net movement of water across the bladder simultaneously with two unidirectional fluxes of urea and observed that the flux of urea was accelerated in the direction of the movement of water while the other was retarded. This observation strongly suggests that urea and water occupy a common channel, a view which is supported by thermodynamic analyses of the permeability of biological membranes for non-electrolyte solutes (Kedem & Katchalsky, 1958).

In contrast to water and urea, which move passively across the membrane, sodium ions are transported actively and energy derived from metabolism is consumed to pump the sodium ions. This active transport can be stimulated by mammalian neurohypophysial hormones and is accompanied by an enhanced metabolism as assessed from oxygen consumption. The metabolic changes, however, are not a direct effect of vasopressin. In preparations in which sodium was removed from the bathing fluid, addition of vasopressin did not produce an increase of oxygen consumption, though the effects of the hormone on transfer of water and urea remained unchanged. According to Civan, Kedem & Leaf (1966) the antidiuretic hormone acts on the permeability barrier to sodium only and not on the transport system of this ion; i.e. it lowers the activation energy for entry of sodium in the membrane.

In an attempt to account for the discrepancies between the passage of water and solute through the toad skin, Andersen & Ussing (1957) postulated the existence of two barriers in series. They suggested the existence of some diffusion barrier, highly permeable to water but almost impermeable to small solutes, under which there is another porous barrier upon which vasopressin would act. Changes in pore size in the deeper barrier, as a result of the action of the antidiuretic hormone, would produce the conditions for bulk flow of water, without affecting the entry of the small solute molecules. This hypothesis of a dual barrier has been supported by Lichtenstein & Leaf (1965, 1966) in experiments in which they used amphotericin B. According to Lampen, Arnow & Safferman (1960) and Lampen, Arnow, Borowska & Laskin (1962) amphotericin B is an antibiotic which interacts with the sterols in cell membranes of micro-organisms; it destroys the mucosal barrier which normally accounts for the low permeability of the tissue to solutes such as potassium, thiourea or chloride, without affecting the tissue characteristics so far as water permeability is concerned. Lichtenstein & Leaf (1966) showed that addition of 5 µg of amphotericin B/ml. to the bathing medium on

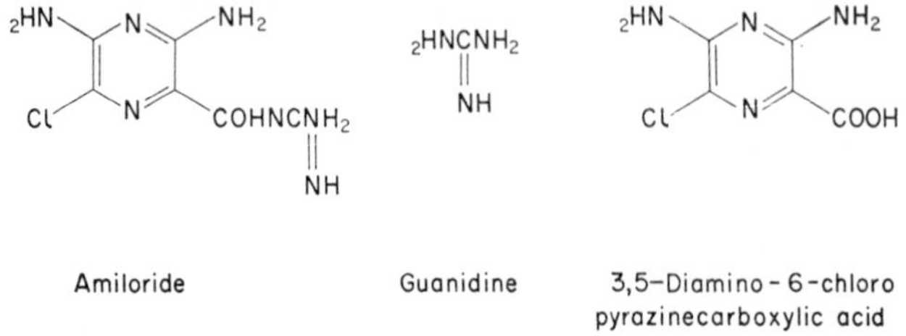

| | Amiloride | Guanidine | 3,5-Diamino-6-chloro pyrazinecarboxylic acid |

FIG. 7.1. Structures of amiloride, guanidine and 3,5-diaminor 6-chloropyrazine-carboxylic acid (from Bentley, 1968a)

the mucosal side of an isolated bladder produced an increase in its permeability to urea, without affecting the movement of water. Subsequent addition of vasopressin (25–50 mu./ml.) had no further effect on the permeability to urea but produced a marked increase in net water transfer.

Recently, Bentley (1968a) used amiloride, a pyrazine diuretic, 3,5-diamino-6-chloropyrazinoylguanidine (Fig. 7.1), a substance

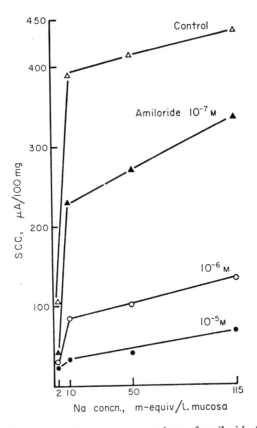

FIG. 7.2. Effects of different concentrations of amiloride (10 min exposure) on the SCC across the toad bladder with the mucosal surface bathed with different concentrations of NaCl. Isotonicity with the serosal Ringer solution was maintained by substituting choline for Na. Each point represents the mean of six different experiments. Δ, control; amiloride: ●, 10^{-5} M; O, 10^{-6} M; ▲, 10^{-7} M. SCC: short-circuit current (from Bentley, 1968a).

which according to Baer, Jones, Spitzer & Russo (1967) reduces sodium transport across the renal tubules (Fig. 7.2). Applied to the mucosal side of an isolated toad bladder in a concentration of 10^{-7} M, amiloride inhibits the effects of vasopressin, of cyclic adenosine monophosphate and of aldosterone, which all increase the transport of sodium and the short-circuit current across the bladder; it has, however, no effect on the transfer of water whether vasopressin is present or not. Furthermore, it does not interfere with the action of amphotericin B (Bentley, 1968b). It would thus appear that the transfer of sodium across the toad bladder takes place in two

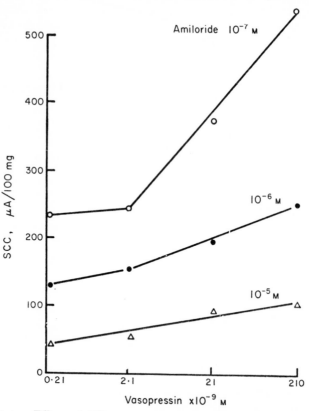

FIG. 7.3. Effects of different concentrations of amiloride on SCC across the toad bladder in the presence of different concentrations of arginine–vasopressin. Each point is the mean of six different experiments. Amiloride: O, 10^{-7} M; ●, 10^{-6} M; Δ, 10^{-5} M. (from Bentley, 1968a).

successive stages: a passive movement across the mucosal boundary into the cell followed by its extrusion against an electrochemical gradient at the serosal side, where, according to Leaf (1960, 1965) the so-called sodium pump is situated. Vasopressin, aldosterone, cyclic adenosine monophosphate and amphotericin B increase the permeability of the mucosal barrier to sodium (Crabbe & De Weer, 1965; Lichtenstein & Leaf, 1965) whereas ouabain inhibits the sodium pump on the serosal side (Herrera, 1966) and reduces the action of amphotericin B. Since amiloride inhibits the actions of vasopressin, aldosterone and cyclic adenosine monophosphate, but not that of amphotericin B, it would appear that amiloride restricts the entry of sodium across the mucosal side of the epithelial cells of the toad bladder without interfering with the transport of water. It is of interest that amphotericin B and amiloride are effective when added to the mucosal side of the toad bladder, in contrast with vasopressin which acts only when added to the serosal side.

Though the 'pore theory' stands as a most satisfactory explanation of the permeability of membranes, it has been criticized on the

TABLE 7.1

Effects of amiloride on the actions of vasopressin, cyclic AMP and amphotericin B on SCC across the toad bladder

	$\mu A/100$ mg bladder			
	Initial	10 min	Diff.	P
I.				
Vasopressin ($2 \cdot 1 \times 10^{-9}$ M)	224	288	$+64 \pm 13$	
Vasopressin + amiloride (10^{-5} M)	27	33	6 ± 2	< 0·01
II.				
Cyclic AMP (2×10^{-3} M)	204	276	$+72 \pm 9$	
Cyclic AMP + amiloride (10^{-5} M)	57	45	-12 ± 6	< 0·001
III.				
Amphotericin B ($1 \cdot 3 \times 10^{-5}$ M)	154	398	$+244 \pm 60$	
Amphotericin B + amiloride (10^{-5} M)	33	411	$+378 \pm 47$	n.s.

Results are given as measured differences $\pm$ s.e. of 6 experiments. The bladder preparations were exposed to the amiloride for 10 min before adding the other compounds (from Bentley, 1968a).

ground that an unstirred layer adjacent to the diffusion barrier could result in a reduction of the estimated coefficient for diffusion permeability (Dainty & House, 1966). This is certainly what appears to happen with thin artificial lipid membranes where the discrepancy between the two coefficients of permeability can be eliminated by stirring. In these membranes net movement of water appears to obtain as a result of free diffusion of water and solubilization in the membrane (Orloff & Handler, 1964). The existence of an unstirred layer would not account, however, for the phenomenon of solvent drag. The phenomenon of solvent drag still remains the most important argument in favour of non-diffusional bulk flow through aqueous channels in biological membranes. If, however, the coefficient of permeability by diffusion of a biological membrane submitted to the action of vasopressin is calculated by measuring the flux of labelled water in the direction of net water movement, the calculated coefficient appears to be too small to account for the observed net flow on the basis of diffusion alone. The presence of an unstirred layer is, therefore, of considerable importance in the interpretation of the mechanism of permeability in complex biological membranes, and in that respect the demonstration by Dainty & House (1966) that the coefficient of permeability can be altered by mere stirring nullifies the calculation of pore size on the basis of Poiseuille's law and the comparison of 'diffusional' and 'osmotic' permeability.

In all experiments using isolated toad bladder, frog skin or renal collecting tubule, the hormone has to be added on the serosal side to be effective. Even large amounts of vasopressin added to the mucosal side are ineffective. This has been observed by every author who has worked in this field. Any attempt to localize the site on which the hormone acts directly or indirectly will help, therefore, to understand its mechanism of action.

Peachey & Rasmussen (1961) studied the histology of preparations of toad bladders in which the mucosal side was exposed to hypotonic solutions. When vasopressin was present they observed a marked swelling of the epithelial cells, which was not visible when the hormone was absent. When, however, the serosal side was bathed with hypotonic solutions there was an almost immediate swelling of the epithelial cells, even in the absence of the hormone. Since vasopressin added to the serosal side induces movement of water when the medium bathing the mucosal side is hypotonic, it would appear that a permeability barrier which normally excludes the water exists at or near the mucosal surface. MacRobbie & Ussing (1961) made similar observations on the frog skin which functionally is analogous to the toad bladder. It will be remembered, however, that in an electron microscopic study of the toad bladder Pak Poy & Bentley (1960) were unable to see any of the structures that 'have been specifically related to water transport in other tissues'.

To come back to the kidney: the earlier studies of Wirz (1956) and of Gottschalk & Mylle (1959) indicated that vasopressin increased the permeability of the distal convoluted tubule of the adult rat. Ullrich, Rumrich & Fuchs (1966) measured the change in the osmolality of fluid perfused through the distal tubule of adult rats *in vivo* and estimated quantitatively the changes in permeability when vasopressin was present. They found that during water diuresis the permeability of the distal tubule of rats was on the average about one third of that observed in the presence of the antidiuretic hormone.

By contrast with the rat, in the dog the antidiuretic hormone has no effect on the permeability of the distal tubules (Clapp & Robinson, 1966). From estimations of inulin concentrations in the distal convoluted tubes of hydropoenic and hydrated dogs, it could be shown that only small amounts of water and solutes were reabsorbed between the early and late portions of this segment, and that the slightly lower osmolality of the fluid observed during a water diuresis could be accounted for by a deficit of urea concentration (Clapp & Robinson, 1966; Bennett *et al.*, 1967).

In both the rat and the dog, and presumably in other mammals, the antidiuretic hormone acts mainly, if not entirely, on the collecting ducts. Grantham & Burg (1966) studied the effects of vasopressin on perfused segments of collecting ducts of rabbits, *in vitro*. They observed that addition of the neurohypophysial hormone to the bathing fluid produced a three-fold increase of the permeability to water, but had no effect when it was added to the liquid in the lumen. The maximum increase of permeability was observed with 25 mu. vasopressin per ml. of the bathing fluid, 60% of the maximum effect being elicited by as little as 5 mu. vasopressin. In contrast with doses used on the isolated toad's bladder (2 u./ml.) which were clearly of a pharmacological order, the amounts of vasopressin used by these workers were almost within the range of concentrations of the antidiuretic hormone found in hydropoenic animals. They found that in contrast with what has been described for the toad bladder and the frog skin, changes in diffusion permeability produced by a difference in osmolality between the lumen and the external medium were of the same order of magnitude as those of net movement of water. In contrast with what has been described for the isolated toad bladder (Maffly, Hays, Lamdin & Leaf, 1960) addition of vasopressin to the perfused distal tubule of the rat (Capek, Rumrich & Ullrich, 1965) and the perfused collecting duct of the rabbit increased the permeability to water but *not* significantly to urea (Grantham & Burg, 1966).

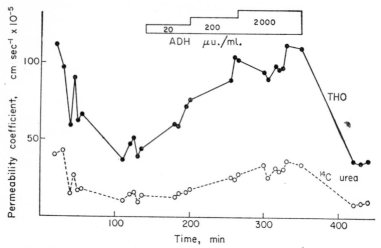

Fig. 7.4. Effects of vasopressin on the permeability coefficient of isolated collecting ducts in rat. Perfusion solution and medium have the same osmolality (515 m-osmoles). Animal not water loaded. THO and urea -^{14}C concentrations were measured and permeability calculated assuming no net movement of water. In other experiments with similar solutions inulin -^{14}C concentrations showed minor changes; perfusion rate 30 nl./min (from Morgan, Sakai & Berliner, 1968).

Morgan, Sakai & Berliner (1968) perfused collecting ducts of an isolated rat papilla with solutions either iso- or hypo-osmotic to the bathing medium. When perfusate and medium had the same composition (515 m.-osmole), the ratio of the osmolality of the fluid in the collecting duct to that of the perfusate was 1·008; it remained unaffected by the addition of 200 μU. vasopressin/ml to the medium. The coefficient of diffusion of water in the absence of antidiuretic hormone was estimated at $53 \pm 4\cdot3$ cm/sec $\times$ 10^{-5}; after addition of vasopressin it rose to $95 \pm 8\cdot5$ cm/sec $\times$ 10^{-5}. In

TABLE 7.2

Comparison of the permeability of cortical and medullary collecting ducts to water and urea

		Cortical collecting ducts*	Medullary collecting ducts
Permeability coefficient for urea, cm sec^{-1} $\times$ 10^{-5}	No ADH	1·05	13·8
	ADH	1·22	20·2
Permeability coefficient for water, cm sec^{-1} $\times$ 10^{-5}	No ADH	37·8	53·0
	ADH	97·1	95·0
Net water movement per unit difference in osmolality, nl cm^{-2} min^{-1} m-osmole^{-1}	No ADH	6·9	4·1
	ADH	23·2	21·0

* From Grantham and Burg (1966)
(from Morgan, Sakai & Berliner, 1968)

the same conditions, the coefficient of permeability for urea rose only from $13\cdot8 \pm 0\cdot79$ to $20\cdot2 \pm 1\cdot3$ cm/sec $\times$ 10^{-5}. When, however, the perfusion fluid (525 m.osmoles) was hypotonic to the medium (735 m-osmoles) there was a unidirectional efflux of water; in the absence of vasopressin the unidirectional movement of water amounted to $36 \pm 4\cdot2$ μl./0·1 cm/min, with a net movement of water of $0\cdot7 \pm 0\cdot12$ ul./0·1 cm/min. After addition of 200 μU. vasopressin/ml., these values rose to $62 \pm 4\cdot0$ and $3\cdot2 \pm 0\cdot42$, respectively. These results confirm the low permeability of the collecting duct to water in the absence of antidiuretic hormone. It is of interest that, in the absence of vasopressin, the permeability of the collecting duct of the rat is of the same order as that of the cortical collecting duct in the rabbit (Grantham & Burg, 1966).

These results are in good agreement with histological studies. Ganote, Grantham, Moses, Burg & Orloff (1968) investigated the ultrastructure of isolated perfused collecting ducts of the rabbit. The perfusion solutions were either isotonic or hypotonic to the external bathing medium. When the perfusing liquid was hypotonic to the medium, addition of vasopressin (25 mu./ml.)

to the latter produced a reversible increase in thickness of the cellular layer, a prominence of cell membranes and the formation of intracellular vacuoles. Examination of the ducts under the

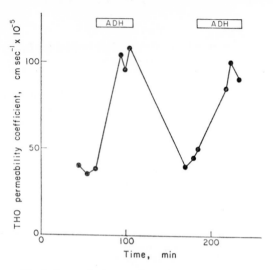

FIG. 7.5. Perfusion solution and medium have the same osmo- lality (515 m-osmoles). The rat was in water diuresis before death. Inulin-^{14}C concentrations indicate no net movement of water. ADH added to give a final concentration of 200 μu./ml. Perfusion rate 30 nl./min (from Morgan *et al.*, 1968).

electron-microscope showed that vasopressin alone, in the absence of an osmotic gradient, had no effect on the ultrastructure. In contrast, when vasopressin was added during a period of high osmotic water transport, they observed prominent dilatation of lateral intercellular spaces, bulging of apical cell membranes into the tubular lumen and formation of intracellular vacuoles, but no modification of the mitochondria. These findings would appear to indicate that vasopressin has no direct effect on the ultrastructure of cells and that the lateral intercellular space is a pathway for os- motically induced transfer of water, while the intracellular changes observed are probably secondary to the flow of water (Figs. 7.6, 7.7 and 7.8). Thus, whereas investigations using epithelial membranes of amphibians had led to the belief that water was flowing directly through the cells via aqueous channels or pores in the apical and basal cell membranes, in the collecting duct of the rabbit this is not so: in the presence of an osmotic gradient and of vasopressin, water is transferred by means of dilatation of intercellular spaces. Though the existence of lateral intercellular spaces had been postulated as an important site of active transport in the rabbit gallbladder and in the rectal papillae of the blowfly (Kaye, Wheeler, Whitlock & Lane, 1966; Diamond & Tormey, 1966; Berridge & Gupta, 1967), it is the first time that such spaces have been recognized in the renal collecting duct of a mammal (Figs. 7.8 and 7.9). Its recognition supports unexpectedly Ginetzinsky's hypothesis (1958). Briefly stated, it is as follows: the intercellular cement of the renal collecting ducts contains hyaluronic acid: during dehydration, following the effect of vasopressin, there is an apocrine secretion of hyaluronidase into the lumen of the ducts which depolymerizes the hyaluronic acid of the intercellular cement and so increases the permeability of the ducts to water. In previous works Ginetzinsky, Broytman & Ivanova (1954) and Ginetzinsky & Ivanova (1958) had shown that hyaluronidase is present in the urine of dehydrated rats and that its concentration is inversely proportional to the rate of urine flow. This was confirmed in other mammals (Ginetzinsky, Krestinskaya, Natochin, Sax & Titova, 1960) and in man (Dicker & Eggleton, 1960, 1961; Cobbin & Dicker, 1962).

Most of the evidence suggesting that the secretion of hyaluronidase may play some role in the mechanism of urine concentration is based on its presence in the urine of hydropoenic mammals. In normal man, hyaluronidase is present whenever the urine is concentrated, the activity of the enzyme being related quantitatively to the degree of antidiuresis. It is absent in the urine of mammals, including man, undergoing a water diuresis (Dicker & Eggleton, 1960; Dicker & Eggleton, 1961). It is absent from the urine of anurans (Ginetzinsky et al., 1960) and that of *Aplodontia rufa* (Dicker & Eggleton, 1964). It is also absent from the urine of patients suffering from nephrogenic diabetes insipidus, a hereditary disease in which the gene responsible is either sex linked or autosomal (Dicker & Eggleton, 1963). Patients with this syndrome do not have an antidiuretic response to the parenteral administration of vasopressin, or to the release of the endogenous hormone. In contrast to normal man, or to patients suffering from diabetes insipidus, administration of vasopressin to people with nephrogenic diabetes insipidus does not produce a secretion of hyaluronidase (Dicker & Eggleton, 1963). Finally, new-born babies, who cannot concentrate their urine (Heller, 1944) even after parenteral administration of vasopressin, do excrete hyaluronidase, whereas infants suffering from nephrogenic diabetes insipidus do not.

Experimental evidence for the possible role of hyaluronidase is rather controversial. Neither Leaf (1960) nor Bentley (1962) could demonstrate any changes in the permeability of the bladders of *Bufo marinus* or *Rana esculenta*, when incubated with hyaluronidase; but both authors used commercial hyaluronidase which is chemically different from the enzyme extracted from the urine (Cobbin & Dicker, 1962; Bollet & Bonner, 1963; Dicker & Elliott, 1963; Dicker & Franklin, 1966). Recently, Natochin & Shakhmatova (1968) reinvestigated the problem and showed that addition of hyaluronidase at pH 5·4 increases the permeability of the urinary bladder of the frog (Fig. 7.10 and Fig. 8.9). The observations of Thorn, Knudsen & Koefoed (1961) that intravenous infusion of large amounts of commercial testicular hyaluronidase into rats or into isolated dog's kidneys produced marked antidiuresis are not relevant since the antidiuretic effect was in all likelihood produced by a fall of the glomerular filtration rate (Cort, 1963; Dicker, 1963). Dicker & Franklin (1966), however, isolated both hyaluronic acid and chondroitin sulphate from the cortex and the medulla of kidneys of pigs, sheep and dogs and confirmed that the urinary hyaluronidase is a different enzyme from that found in other tissues. It effectively depolymerizes the mucopolysaccharides from the kidney. It may be of interest to mention that the depolymerization of the hyaluronic acid of the intercellular cement of renal cells would lead to a liberation of calcium. The observation that in dogs and in man antidiuresis is accompanied by an increased excretion of calcium may, therefore, be of some importance (Thorn, 1960; Dicker & Eggleton, 1961).

Though the 'hyaluronidase' theory has been criticized on histological grounds by Heller & Lojda (1960), Breddy, Cooper & Boss (1961) and Boss, Breddy & Cooper (1961), these criticisms may have lost some of their weight since the new evidence provided by Ganote *et al.* (1968), and by Natochin & Shakhmatova (1968).

Clearly, more work is needed in this field. The question as to how the antidiuretic hormone acts on the nephron is still awaiting

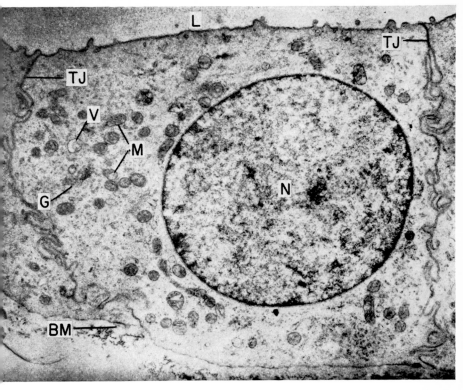

FIG. 7.6. Lining cell of a tubule relatively impermeable to water (Period II); hypotonic
fusion. A few microvilli project into the tubular lumen (L). Adjacent cells are joined by
tight junctional complex near the lumen (TJ). The lateral cell membranes have numerous
terdigitating folds. N, nucleus; M, mitochondria; V, vacuole; G, Golgi region; BM,
asement membrane. × 12,500 (from Ganote, Grantham, Moses, Burg & Orloff, 1968).

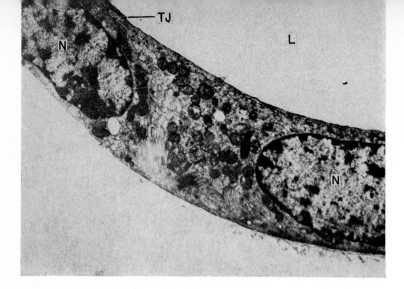

FIG. 7.7. Vasopressin-treated tubule perfused with isotonic solution. There is no swelling of the cells nor dilatation of the lateral intercellular spaces. Intercalated cell on the left lining cell on the right. L, tubule lumen; TJ, tight junction; N, nucleus. × 11,000 (from Ganote et al., 1968).

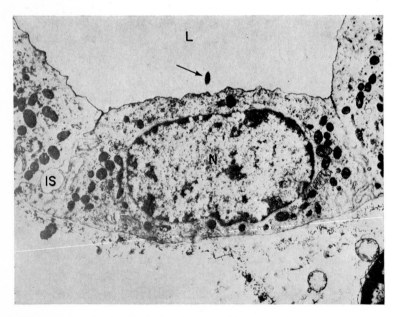

FIG. 7.8. Lining cells of a freshly isolated tubule (Period I); hypotonic infusion. There moderate dilatation of the inter-cellular space on the left (IS), but not on the right. The cell bulges slightly into the tubular lumen (L). A portion of a cilium is seen projecting into the lumen (arrow). N, nucleus. × 12,000, (from Ganote et al., 1968).

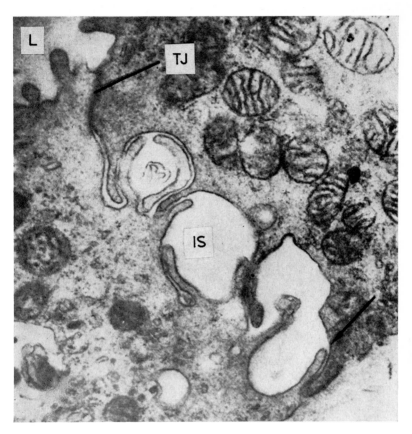

FIG. 7.9. Intercellular space (IS) of vasopressin-treated tubule highly permeable to water (Period III); hypotonic infusion. The tight junction is unaltered (TJ). The intercellular space is dilated in its midportion but narrows abruptly at the base of the cells where the lateral membranes remain closely apposed (arrow). L, tubular lumen. × 20,000 (from Ganote *et al.*, 1968).

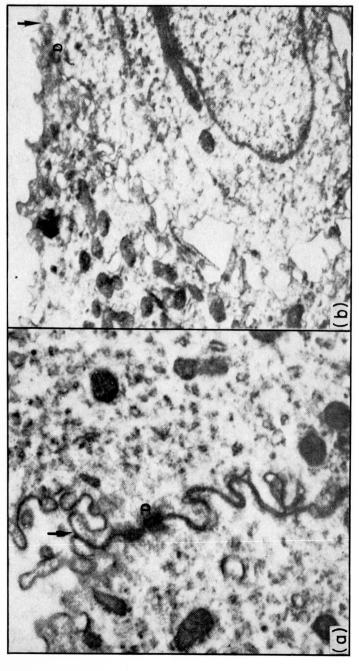

Fig. 7.10. Changes of structure of intercellular space in frog urinary bladder epithelium under the influence of vasopressin. (a) Control; (b) Following the addition of 1 mu./ml. vasopressin (the intercellular space is enlarged). The arrow shows the place of connection of two neighbouring cells; D, desmosome. × 34,000 (from Natochin & Shakhmatova, 1968).

its answer. A better knowledge of the diffusion barriers, their structure and their biochemical properties is still required. It may be even that the present views and theories on the structure and functions of membranes of anurans, however interesting, are restrictive in their interpretation and impede the work of an essentially different nature on the kidneys of mammals.

8

MODE OF ACTION OF THE
ANTIDIURETIC HORMONE

*'I fail to see how we can continue to refer natural functions to the
smallness or largeness of channels, or any other similar hypothesis.'*
Galen (AD 130–200)

WHEN the antidiuretic hormone is released into the blood stream,
or injected intravenously into an animal, about half of its activity
reaches the kidneys, while the other half is destroyed by the liver
(Heller & Urban, 1935; Ginsburg & Heller, 1953; Dicker, 1954).
Of the amount of antidiuretic hormone that reaches the kidney,
some is excreted in the urine (see: Lauson, 1967). But, is the
antidiuretic activity found in the urine that of vasopressin or of a
modified form of vasopressin? According to Heller (1953) and to
Mayer (1960) it is identical with that of vasopressin. Dicker &
Nunn (1957), however, suggested it might be a mixture of vasopressin and of a modified form of the hormone. Aroskar, Chan,
Stouffer, Schneider, Murti & Du Vigneaud (1964) injecting tritium-
labelled oxytocin intravenously into an animal showed that the
oxytocic activity excreted into the urine was a mixture of unchanged
oxytocin and of at least two metabolic products also containing the
tritium label. How much vasopressin is excreted in the urine? From
investigations in which the urinary excretion of exogenous vasopressin was expressed as a percentage of doses administered, it will
be seen that for doses ranging from 50 to 1,000,000 μU./kg, the
average excretion amounted to: 12% in rats (Heller, 1952;
Ginsburg & Heller, 1953; Ginsburg, 1954; Dicker & Nunn, 1957;
Sawyer, 1963; Smith & Thorn, 1965): 28% in cats (Jones &
Schlapp, 1936; Larson, 1938): 25% in dogs (Larson, 1938;
O'Connor, 1950; Lauson, Bocanegra & Beuzeville, 1965; Thorn
& Smith, 1965; Harvey, Jones & Lee 1967); and about 10% in
man (Orr & Snaith, 1959; Dicker & Eggleton, 1960; Czaczkes &

Kleeman, 1964). Since about half only of the administered vaso-pressin reaches the kidneys, approximately 30% of the vasopressin entering the renal arteries is excreted in the urine. How does vaso-pressin enter the urine? Results from stop-flow studies in dogs injected with large doses of tritiated arginine–vasopressin suggest that the excretion of vasopressin is by glomerular filtration only (Towbin & Ferrell, 1963; Sawyer, 1963; Lauson et al., 1965). This, however, does not agree with findings by Thorn & Silver (1957), Smith & Thorn (1965), Tata, Heller & Gauer (1965), Ahmed, George, Gonzalez-Auvert & Dingman) (1967) and Harvey et al. (1967), according to whom vasopressin circulates in blood bound to a protein, or with observations by Heller (1937, 1957) who showed that the rate of dialysis through a cellophane membrane was markedly slower when vasopressin was mixed with blood plasma than when it was in saline solution. Lauson (1967), who reviewed the question of the physical state of vasopressin in the blood, stated that 'data on the extent to which endogenous and exogenous ADH is bound to plasma proteins are conflicting, but the weight of evi-dence indicates that in all the species studied, much, most or even all of the hormone circulates in the free peptide form'. If vaso-pressin, with a molecular weight of just over 1000, circulates as a free peptide, there is every likelihood that it is first filtered by the glomeruli, and then reabsorbed by the tubules (Fig. 8.1).

Assuming that the vasopressin which appears in the urine is that which has escaped reabsorption, what would be its function? From studies on the isolated toad bladder or frog skin, vaso-pressin has an effect on the permeability of the membrane only when added to the serosal, i.e. outer side. Grantham & Burg (1966), and Morgan et al. (1968) reached the same conclusion for the renal collecting duct: to be active vasopressin had to be added to the medium bathing the outside of the duct. Since the anti-diuretic effect obtains essentially when vasopressin reaches the late portions of the distal tubule and of the collecting duct by way of blood vessels, it can be assumed that the amount of antidiuretic activity excreted in the urine has little physiological function. Moreover, since all the blood vessels in the renal medulla and those of the distal tubules originate from the glomerular efferent arterioles, it is tempting to speculate that the amounts of vaso-pressin needed to produce an antidiuretic effect may ultimately be regulated by the state of constriction of the efferent arterioles.

Whether the hormone circulates free or bound it will act upon selective receptor sites. In the anuran, the antidiuretic hormone is arginine[8]–vasotocin, an analogue of vasopressin. Morel & Jard (1963) showed that the intravascular injections of small amounts of the order of 0·01–0·02 µ/100 g of either arginine[8]–vasotocin or its

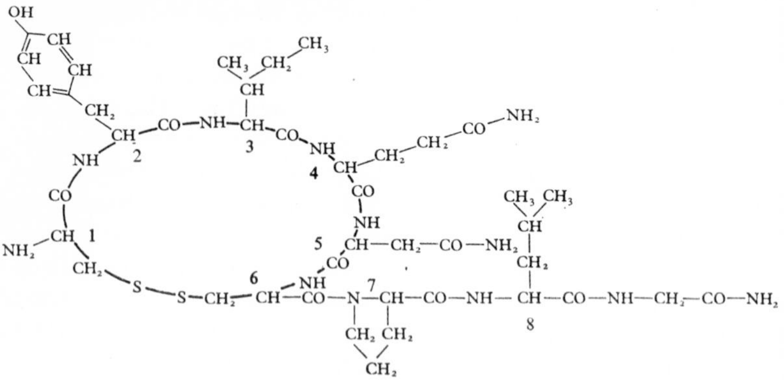

The structure of oxytocin

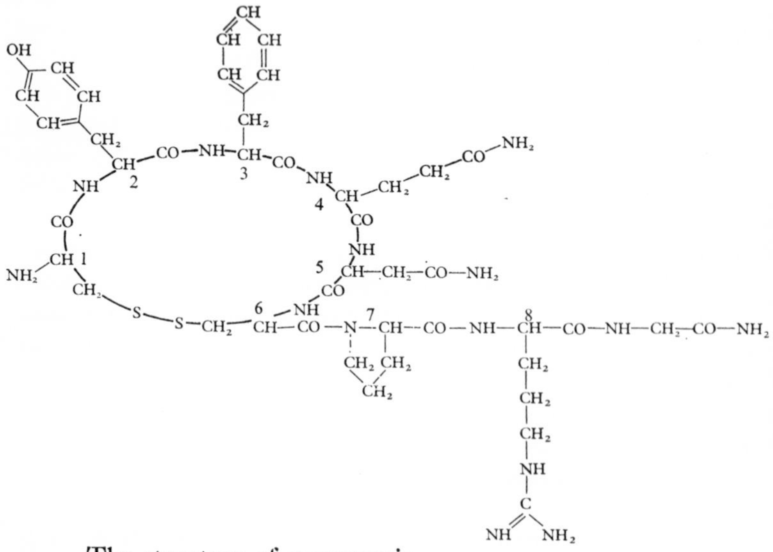

The structure of vasopressin

FIG. 8.1

lysine derivative increase the rate of tubular water and sodium reabsorption in the frog, whereas oxytocin and vasopressin not only were devoid of these effects, but oxytocin was an inhibitor of vasotocin. The experiments were performed on large male *Rana esculenta* (weight *c.* 100 g) in which the rate of glomerular filtration, the free water, the osmolar, the sodium and the potassium clearances were estimated. Intra-arterial administration of arginine[8]– and of lysine[8]–vasotocin produced a marked decrease, of the order of 35% of the free-water clearance, and some decrease of sodium clearance. Injections of oxytocin, deamino-oxytocin, iso-leucine[8], or valine[8]–oxytocin had no such effects. Though these analogues were all inactive, they inhibited almost completely the effect of subsequent injections of lysine[8]– or arginine[8]–vasotocin. In contrast, neither vasopressin nor its analogues oxypressin or Phe[2]–Phe[3]–oxytocin exhibited an inhibitory effect against vaso-tocin (Table 8.1).

From these results Morel & Jard concluded that those poly-peptides which have in their molecule a ring structure identical with, or at least closely related to, that of vasotocin are inhibitor and act very likely by competitive fixation on a receptor site; whereas those compounds with a ring different from that of vaso-tocin, even though their side chains are identical, are neither active nor inhibitory because they are not bound by the receptor; further, though it is the cyclic structure of the molecule which combines with the receptor, it is its side chain that determines the specific activity of the polypeptide, i.e. its ability to change the permea-bility of the nephron to water.

Evidence for competitive inhibition involving 'receptors' has also been suggested for mammals. For instance, in rats, the pressor response to arginine[8]–vasopressin can be inhibited by large doses of oxytocin (Ressler & Rachelle, 1958) and in rabbits and dogs by a synthetic peptide di-carbobenzoxy-L-cystinyl-di-tyrosine-ethyl ester (Ishida & Hara, 1964). Likewise, the inactivation of arginine[8]–vasopressin by rat kidney slices can be prevented by addition to the incubation medium of chlormercuribenzoate (Dicker & Greenbaum, 1958) or oxytocin (Smith & Sachs, 1961). No inhibition, however, could be demonstrated on the toad bladder, between oxytocin and 2-O-methyltyrosine derivative of oxytocin (Rasmussen & Schwartz, 1964) though such a competitive antagonism had been shown to exist on the rat uterus (Rudinger

TABLE 8.1

Correlation between chemical structure and inhibitory property of some polypeptides (after Morel & Jard, 1963)

Name and Amino Acid Sequence	Radicals substituted in Vasotocin molecule				Antidiuretic activity	Inhibitory action against vasotoc[in]
	position 1	position 2	position 3	position 8		
Lysine-Vasotocin 1 2 3 8 Cys-Tyr-Ileu-Glu(NH₂)-Asp(NH₂)-Cys-Pro-Lys-Gly(NH₂)	SH CH₂ CH-NH₂	OH ⬡ CH₂	CH₃ CH₂ CH-CH₃	NH₂ (CH₂)₄	+	
Arginine-Vasotocin Cys-Tyr-Ileu-Glu(NH₂)-Asp(NH₂)-Cys-Pro-Arg-Gly(NH₂)				NH₂ C=NH NH (CH₂)₃	+	
Lysine-Vasopressin Cys-Tyr-Phe-Glu(NH₂)-Asp(NH₂)-Cys-Pro-Lys-Gly(NH₂)			⬡ CH₂		none	none
Oxypressin Cys-Tyr-Phe-Glu(NH₂)-Asp(NH₂)-Cys-Pro-Leu-Gly(NH₂)			⬡ CH₂	CH₃ CH-CH₃ CH₂	none	none
Phe^{2,3}Lys^{8}-Oxytocin Cys-Phe-Phe-Glu(NH₂)-Asp(NH₂)-Cys-Pro-Lys-Gly(NH₂)		⬡ CH₂	⬡ CH₂		none	none
Oxytocin Cys-Tyr-Ileu-Glu(NH₂)-Asp(NH₂)-Cys-Pro-Leu-Gly(NH₂)				CH₃ CH-CH₃ CH₂	none	+
Desamino-Oxytocin β-merc-prop-ac-Tyr-Ileu-Glu(NH₂)-Asp(NH₂)-Cys-Pro-Leu-Gly(NH₂)	SH CH₂ CH₂			CH₃ CH-CH₃ CH₂	none	+
Ileu^{8}-Oxytocin Cys-Tyr-Ileu-Glu(NH₂)-Asp(NH₂)-Cys-Pro-Ileu-Gly(NH₂)				CH₃ CH₂ CH-CH₃	none	+
Val^{3}-Oxytocin Cys-Tyr-Val-Glu(NH₂)-Asp(NH₂)-Cys-Pro-Leu-Gly(NH₂)			CH₃ CH-CH₃	CH₃ CH-CH₃ CH₂	none	+.

& Jost, 1964*a*). Also relevant is the observation that extracts of the pituitary gland of rats affected by hereditary diabetes insipidus inhibit the antidiuretic response to vasopressin (Sawyer & Valtin, 1965). Since the neural lobe of the rats suffering from diabetes insipidus contain oxytocin only, it has been suggested that this inhibition might be due to oxytocin. This, however, is not probable since intravenous administration of oxytocin fails to have an inhibitory effect.

In the kidneys of mammals, there is evidence indicating that the hormone has to be absorbed before it can exert its antidiuretic action. Heller & Urban (1935), Fromageot & Maier-Hüser (1951), Maier-Hüser, Clauser, Fromageot & Plongeron (1953) all have shown that vasopressin is bound on tissues. It is bound by homogenates from kidney, liver, spleen and duodenum; it is not bound by muscles (Dicker & Greenbaum, 1956), nor by erythrocytes (Heller & Zaidi, 1957; Bocanegra & Lauson, 1961). Tissues which bind vasopressin inactivate it, the others do not (Dicker & Greenbaum, 1956). It is of interest that in patients suffering from nephrogenic diabetes insipidus in whom sites of binding are supposed to be either congenitally absent, deficient or abnormal (Orloff & Burg, 1960; Cutler, Kleeman, Maxwell & Dowling, 1962) more than 50% of intravenously injected vasopressin was excreted in the urine, which suggests that in these patients none of the vasopressin that reached the kidneys had been inactivated (Dicker & Eggleton, 1960).

More than twenty-five years ago van Dyke, Chow, Greep & Rothen (1942) had shown that the antidiuretic activity of vasopressin is abolished by cleavage of the ring at the —S—S— link, a fact which has been confirmed by other research workers. Dicker & Greenbaum (1958) observed that incubation of vasopressin with cysteine and glutathione reduced its antidiuretic activity, whereas cystine left it unchanged. They further showed that the inactivation of vasopressin by the particle-free supernatant of kidney homogenates was produced by an enzyme, possibly acting on the —S—S— link of the molecule, reducing it to —SH. Since the enzyme could be activated by compounds like cysteine or glutathione, containing an —SH— group, they concluded that the enzyme is an —SH enzyme with maximum activity in the —SH form. This interpretation agreed with the findings of Cafruny, Carhart & Farah (1957) who investigated the effects of various hormones on the concentration of thiols in kidney cells and found that vasopressin produced a decrease of sulphydryl groups in the distal convoluted tubes. No change in the concentration of thiols was observed with another disulphide hormone, the growth hormone, or with hormones such as thyroxin or thyrotrophin.

Rasmussen, Schwartz, Schoessler & Hochster (1960), using the amphibian bladder, investigated the mode of action of a number of sulphydryl reagents which all inhibited the effect of vasopressin. Though vasopressin was effective only when added to the serosal (outer) side of the bladder, the other sulphydryl compounds were active when added either to the serosal or the mucosal side. When added in concentrations of 1×10^{-4} to 1×10^{-5} M to the mucosal surface, sulphydryl compounds induced a change of permeability which was qualitatively similar to that of vasopressin added to the serosal surface, but in contrast with the action of vasopressin it was irreversible. This led them to believe that the primary interactions between vasopressin and its receptor in the bladder involves an interchange reaction between disulphide and sulphydryl (Rasmussen, Schwartz, Young & Marc Aurele, 1963).

This view has been supported by Fong, Schwartz, Popenoe, Silver & Schoessler (1959) who postulated that the interaction of vasopressin with 'receptors' in the kidney might involve the formation of a covalent bond as the result of an exchange reaction between thiol and disulphide groups. This hypothesis was confirmed in an investigation in which tritiated arginine[8]–vasopressin [3]HAVP was injected into rats. Ten minutes after the injection, i.e. at the peak of the antidiuretic effect, the animals were killed and the kidneys dropped into liquid nitrogen. They were then homogenized with ice saturated with N-phenylmaleimide to bind sulphydryl groups. After various treatments, fractions of the kidney proteins were shaken with either cysteine, sodium thioglycollate or β-mercaptoethylamine and finally prepared for tritium analysis. The result of these experiments indicated the existence of a sulphur—sulphur bond which was interpreted as representing the interaction of the hormone and the receptor (Fong, Silver, Christman & Schwartz, 1960; Schwartz, Rasmussen, Schoessler, Silver & Fong, 1960).

This type of experiment was extended by Schwartz, Rasmussen, Livingston & Marc-Aurele (1964) who injected into a renal artery or a jugular vein of a rat four to fifty millimicrograms of

^{3}H–arginine–vasopressin with a specific radioactivity of 426 μc/mg. At the appropriate time after the injection of the labelled vasopressin, the kidneys were perfused *in situ* with 0·9% NaCl solution containing sulphydryl-blocking reagents; they were then removed, fixed by immersion in boiling absolute alcohol containing 10^{-3}M N–ethylmaleimide, homogenized, washed free from any radioactivity bound by electrovalency and then treated with a thiol or sulphite reagent to release any disulphide-bound radioactivity from the sediment. In four experiments, rats were killed 5 to 10 minutes after the injection of the tritiated hormone, i.e. at the peak of the antidiuresis; in four more experiments they were killed only after the antidiuresis had subsided and the urine flow was back to its pre-injection rate. In the experiments in which the kidneys were removed at the peak of the antidiuresis the disulphide-bound radioactivity was found to give an average of 64·3 (range 55·0 to 77·5) counts/min per gram kidney, whereas in those where full diuresis had been resumed, the average count was 3·3 (range 1·8 to 7·1) per minute per gram kidney. The experiments were then repeated with tritiated oxytocin instead of vasopressin. First oxytocin was injected in a dosage equivalent to the amount of vasopressin that produced a maximum antidiuretic effect (0·5 mμg). This, however, as expected, had no effect on the diuresis. When the dose of tritiated oxytocin was increased hundred-fold, a significant antidiuretic response was observed. In the first series, with small amounts of oxytocin the release of disulphide-bound activity averaged 2·9 counts/min per gram kidney only, whereas in the other series the counts averaged 43·3 per minute per gram kidney. It would appear, therefore, that there is a close correlation between the dosage required to produce a specific physiological effect and a measurable binding of the hormone, and that there is a high degree of specificity of molecular structure for the formation of mixed disulphides between hormones and renal tissue.

Further evidence of the importance of disulphide bridges came from investigations by Lehninger and Neubert (1961) who found that vasopressin, oxytocin and insulin, all of which contain disulphide bridges, are potent swelling agents of liver mitochondria and that their mode of action resembles that of simple disulphides such as oxidized glutathione or cystamine. The hormones, however, were some 100 times more active mole for mole than other disulphide compounds. This quantitative difference suggests that

E

the amino sequence and the conformation of peptide chain are responsible for the enhanced swelling action of the disulphide group. Greenbaum & Dicker (1963a, b) incubated mitochondria from the cortex and from the medulla of dog's kidneys with oxytocin, lysine[8]– and arginine[8]–vasopressins. The rate of water

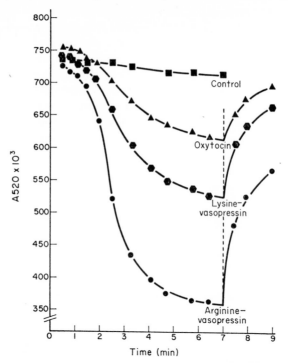

FIG. 8.2. The effect of arginine–vasopressin (●—●), lysine–vasopressin (●—●) and oxytocin (▲—▲) on the swelling of rat-liver mitochondria. ATP (ATP, 5 mM; MgCl₂, 5 mM; bovine serum albumin 0·2 mg/ml. final concentration) was added at the time marked by the dotted line. Medium: 0·125 M KCl–0·02 M Tris. Temperature, 18° C. The swelling of the mitochondria was followed by measuring the light absorption at 520 mμ (from Greenbaum & Dicker, 1963a).

uptake by the mitochondria was estimated by following their swelling as measured by changes in light absorption. They found that mitochondria from the renal medulla were much more sensitive to the presence of the hormones than those from the cortex, and that arginine[8]–vasopressin was the most potent hormone and oxytocin the least (Fig. 8.2). The swelling of the mitochondria could be reversed by addition of ATP. It is interesting that the basicity of the amino acid in position 8 in the molecule of the neurohypophysial hormones determines the amount of water that isolated mitochondria take up as well as the degree by which the permeability of the cells in the distal part of the nephron changes. This then reinforces the views expressed by Morel & Jard (1963) that, whereas it is the cyclic structure of the molecule that combines with the receptor, it is the amino acids in the side chain that are responsible for the change of permeability of membranes. One can therefore postulate that the interchange reactions involved in the formation of a hormone-receptor disulphide bond serve as a physiological trigger to the chain of events leading eventually to changes in the permeability of the membrane.

This led Fong *et al.* (1960) to suggest as a hypothesis the following mechanism for the action of the antidiuretic hormone: the hormone is attracted to its receptor site by electrostatic interactions operating between the positively charged groups of the hormone and the negatively charged group of the receptor. The tyrosyl–hydroxyl group and amide groups of glutamine, asparagine and glycinamide of the molecule of vasopressin might be prominent in providing the attractive force. The ensuing reactions between attractive and repulsive forces bring about the right alignment of the hormone with its receptor. This is followed by the thiol–disulphide exchange reaction, which consists in an attack of the mercaptide ion of the receptor on the disulphide group of the hormone producing a hormone-receptor disulphide. This now gives rise to a series of sulphydryl–disulphide reactions which are responsible for alterations of the structure of membrane proteins, which eventually bring about changes in the protein components of the diffusion barrier and allow an increase in the flux of water through what is likely to be a 'loosened' membrane (Fong *et al.*, 1960). Eventually the reaction ends by a cleavage of the hormone-receptor disulphide bond, possibly of the nature suggested by Dicker & Greenbaum (1958). This reaction, in which the sulphydryl group of the receptor is regenerated, restores the membrane to its original state.

This theory, if correct, would not be restricted to the action of neurohypophysial hormones but could be extended to that of insulin, whose prime function is to alter the permeability of certain membranes to sugars. In common with vasopressin, insulin can be inactivated by partial reduction of the intra-chain disulphide bond of its molecule, which clearly suggests a thiol–disulphide exchange similar to that postulated for the antidiuretic hormone. In 1964, however, Rudinger & Jost synthesized a biologically active analogue of oxytocin in which one sulphur atom of the disulphide bridge of deamino-oxytocin had been replaced by a methylene group, and which therefore did not contain a disulphide group (Fig. 8.3). The same year Schwartz, Rasmussen & Rudinger (1964) reported

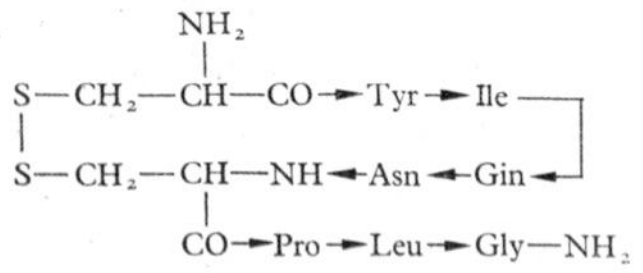

$$NH_2$$
$$S—CH_2—CH—CO \rightarrow Tyr \rightarrow Ile —$$
$$S—CH_2—CH—NH \leftarrow Asn \leftarrow Gin \leftarrow$$
$$CO \rightarrow Pro \rightarrow Leu \rightarrow Gly—NH_2$$

oxytocin

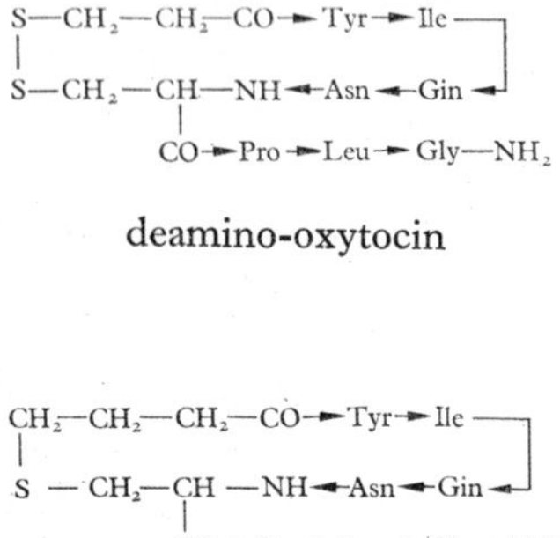

$$S—CH_2—CH_2—CO \rightarrow Tyr \rightarrow Ile —$$
$$S—CH_2—CH—NH \leftarrow Asn \leftarrow Gin \leftarrow$$
$$CO \rightarrow Pro \rightarrow Leu \rightarrow Gly—NH_2$$

deamino-oxytocin

$$CH_2—CH_2—CH_2—CO \rightarrow Tyr \rightarrow Ile —$$
$$S — CH_2—CH —NH \leftarrow Asn \leftarrow Gin \leftarrow$$
$$CO \rightarrow Pro \rightarrow Leu \rightarrow Gly—NH_2$$

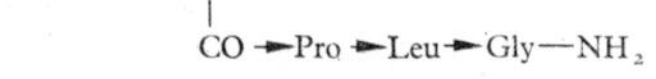

Monocarba analogue of deamino-oxytocin

$$CH_2—CH_2—CH_2—CO \rightarrow Tyr \rightarrow Ile —$$
$$CH_2—CH_2—CH —NH \leftarrow Asn \leftarrow Gin \leftarrow$$
$$CO \rightarrow Pro \rightarrow Leu \rightarrow Gly—NH_2$$

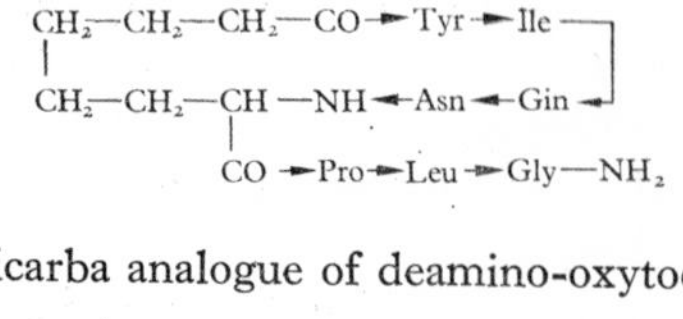

Dicarba analogue of deamino-oxytocin

FIG. 8.3. Schematic representation of the molecular structure of oxytocin and the mono- and dicarba- analogues.

that three other synthetic analogues of oxytocin without a disulphide bridge showed oxytocin-like activity in a number of biological preparations, including the isolated toad bladder, but that their effects were smaller than those elicited by analogues with a disulphide bridge. Finally, Pliska, Rudinger, Dausa & Cort (1968) synthesized two analogues of deamino-oxytocin, with one and both sulphurs in the 1-Cys to 6-Cys disulphide bridge replaced with CH_2 groups. These compounds were tested on the short-circuit current on the frog-skin preparation and on the water-loaded alcohol-anaesthetized rat. In both assays activity was present, although with decreased potency, and—most important—the duration of the effect was the same as that with oxytocin itself. Since it is known that even slight structural changes of the molecule may result in loss of potency, it is not surprising that the potency of analogues with methylene groups was not fully equivalent to compounds with sulphur in this position. But from the observation that the effects of the two analogues had a time course similar to that of oxytocin, it must be accepted that the disulphide reduction–aminopeptidase degradation sequence observed in tissue preparations is unlikely to represent the main pathway of hormone inactivation (Walter, Rudinger & Schwartz, 1967). If enzymic degradation plays a role in limiting the duration of action of these polypeptides, there must be points of attack on the molecule of the hormone other than the disulphide bond. In 1960, Dicker & Greenbaum had reported that renal enzymes can attack the molecule at the site of linkage of the 3 amides, glycine-amide, asparagine and glutamine. In view of the fact that kidneys are known to be a rich source of such amide-splitting enzymes as glutaminase and arginase, this possibility cannot be overlooked (Dicker, 1960).

It may be of interest to mention that more than 200 analogues and homologues of neurohypophysial hormones have been prepared and tested for their activities. Though it is impossible to give any details here certain interesting considerations seem to have emerged from these investigations. The size of the cyclic moiety seems to be optimal; enlargement or reduction of it is deleterious to the oxytocin-like activities. Shortening of the peptide side-chain decreases the oxytocic activity of analogues. Many modifications of the natural structures are still compatible with considerable biological activities. The L configuration of the

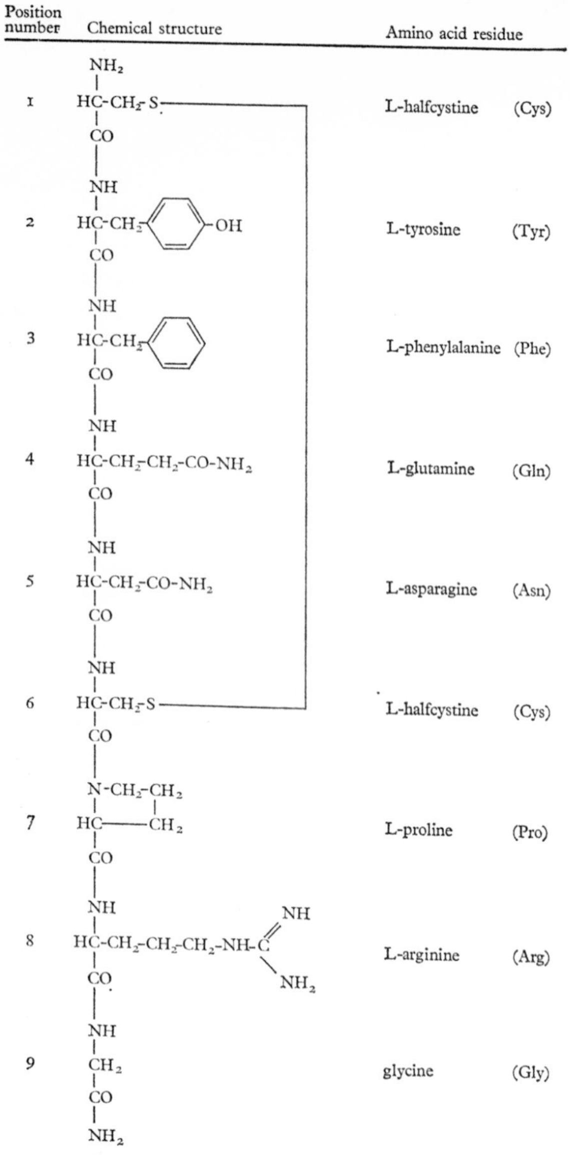

Position number	Chemical structure	Amino acid residue	
1	NH$_2$ | HC-CH$_2$-S—— | CO	L-halfcystine	(Cys)
2	NH | HC-CH$_2$-⬡-OH | CO	L-tyrosine	(Tyr)
3	NH | HC-CH$_2$-⬡ | CO	L-phenylalanine	(Phe)
4	NH | HC-CH$_2$-CH$_2$-CO-NH$_2$ | CO	L-glutamine	(Gln)
5	NH | HC-CH$_2$-CO-NH$_2$ | CO	L-asparagine	(Asn)
6	NH | HC-CH$_2$-S—— | CO	L-halfcystine	(Cys)
7	N-CH$_2$-CH$_2$ | | HC———CH$_2$ | CO	L-proline	(Pro)
8	NH NH | ⫽ HC-CH$_2$-CH$_2$-CH$_2$-NH-C | \\ CO NH$_2$	L-arginine	(Arg)
9	NH | CH$_2$ | CO | NH$_2$	glycine	(Gly)

FIG. 8.4. Developed chemical formula of vasopressin.

Position number	Chemical structure	Amino acid residue	
1	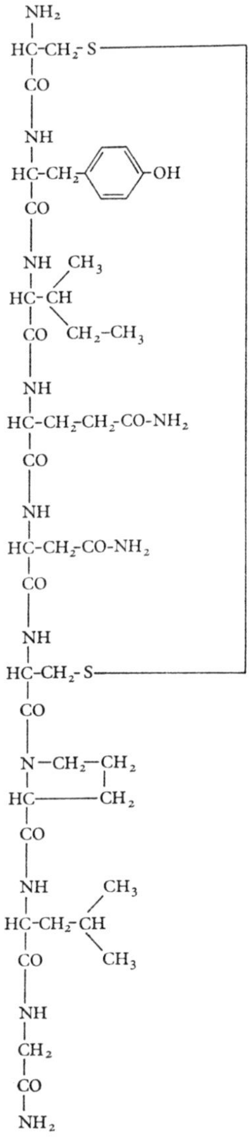	L-halfcystine	(Cys)
2		L-tyrosine	(Tyr)
3		L-isoleucine	(Ile)
4		L-glutamine	(Gln)
5		L-asparagine	(Asn)
6		L-halfcystine	(Cys)
7		L-proline	(Pro)
8		L-leucine	(Leu)
9		glycine	(Gly)

FIG. 8.5. Developed chemical formula of oxytocin.

amino-acid residues does not appear to be indispensable for bio-logical activity. Finally, neither the free amino group in position 1 nor the phenolic–hydroxyl group in position 2, nor the disulphide bond in positions 1 and 6 are essential. On the other hand, a basic group in position 8 clearly favours vasopressin-like activity. Of the three carboxamide group in positions 4, 5 and 9, the one in position 5 is of particular importance for biological activity (Berde, 1968; Berde & Boissonnas, 1968).

In tissues such as toad bladder or frog skin, vasopressin stimulates glycogenolysis and oxygen consumption (Leaf & Dempsey, 1960; Orloff & Handler, 1964; Bentley, 1965). Examination of the metabolic effects of neurohypophysial hormones using metabolic inhibitors has, however, yielded conflicting results. Virtually all inhibitors studied interfere with sodium

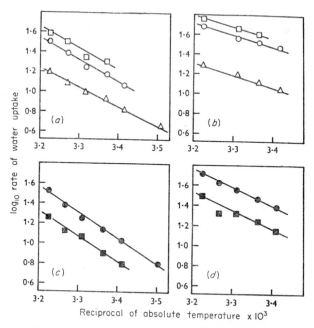

FIG. 8.6. Arrhenius plots of logarithm of water uptake across the skin (μl./cm^2/hr) for toads kept in various solutions at temperatures between 12 and 37°C. (a) and (c) before vasopressin; (b) and (d) after vasopressin (4 m-u./g). ●—●, water; ▦—▦, 73 m-osmolar sucrose; □—□, 51 m-osmolar NaCl; O—O, 97 m-osmolar NaCl; △—△ 191 m-osmolar NaCl (Dicker & Elliott, 1967)

transport and the short-circuit current response to the hormones (Bentley, 1966; Handler, Petersen & Orloff, 1966). But, according to Rasmussen, *et al.* (1960), metabolic inhibitors have no effect on the hydro-osmotic response to vasopressin, which would suggest that the increase in size of the aqueous channels induced by vasopressin does not require energy and is independent of oxidative mechanisms of the cells. Dicker & Elliott (1967), however, have shown that administration of vasopressin to the toad, *Bufo melanostictus*, reduces the activation energy, which indirectly supports the suggestion previously made by Koefoed–Johnsen &

TABLE 8.6

Values of activation energy derived from Arrhenius equation obtained from Fig. 8.6

Bathing solution	Treatment	Concentration (m-osmole/l.)	Calculated slope	Estimated activation energy (cal.)
Water	—	—	2·56	12,000
Water	Vasopressin	—	1·75	8,000
Sucrose solution	—	73	2·50	12,000
Sucrose solution	Vasopressin	73	1·85	8,000
NaCl solution	—	191	1·88 ⎫	
		97	2·26 ⎬ 2·06	9,000
		51	2·04 ⎭	
NaCl solution	Vasopressin	191	1·15 ⎫	
		97	1·03 ⎬ 1·08	5,000
		51	0·98 ⎭	

All injections of vasopressin were 4 m-u./g.
(Dicker & Elliott, 1967)

Ussing (1963) (Fig. 8.6 and Table 8.2). Recently, Orloff & Handler (1967) studied the rate at which glycogenolysis takes place in toad bladder in the absence and presence of vasopressin and found no difference in the concentration of high-energy phosphate compounds such as creatine phosphate, ADP or ATP. They observed, however, changes in the concentration of glycogenolytic intermediates such as phosphofructokinase, pyruvate kinase and phosphorylase. The presence of sodium in the Ringer's solution used may play a critical role in eliciting these metabolic changes (Bentley, 1966). In this respect, it should be recalled that although vasopressin increases the activity of phosphorylase in homogenates of toad bladder incubated in a sodium-free medium, according to Handler & Orloff (1963) and Orloff and Handler (1967) it has no effect on the oxygen consumption and glycogenolysis in the intact animal.

These metabolic effects of vasopressin are not restricted to its action on the kidneys or the toad bladder. Injections of vasopressin into the adrenal artery of a dog produce a release of cortisol, in a manner analogous to ACTH and injections of vasopressin into the portal vein produce a release of glucose from the liver, an effect similar to that of glucagon or adrenaline (Bergen, Sullivan, Hilton, Willis & van Itallie, 1960). Such effects suggest that whatever the ultimate mechanism of vasopressin, its action might be mediated by at least one other substance. Already in 1957, Haynes & Berthet and three years later Sutherland & Rall (1960) proposed that a variety of hormones exert their effects through the action of cyclic adenosine $3',5'$-monophosphate (AMP). They showed that ACTH, which stimulates the release of cortisol from the adrenal glands, increases the concentration of cyclic AMP in the tissue, and that adrenaline and glucagon, which cause the liberation of glucose from the liver, also increase the intrahepatic formation of cyclic AMP. Furthermore, cyclic AMP mimics the action of ACTH on the adrenal gland, and the effect of glucagon and adrenaline on the liver. In the light of these results Orloff & Handler (1964) suggested that vasopressin stimulates the production and/or the accumulation of cyclic AMP in both toad bladder and mammalian kidney, the cyclic adenosine $3'5'$-monophosphate being ultimately responsible for the modification of the permeability of these tissues to water. According to their views, very concisely expressed, vaso-pressin accelerates the normal conversion of ATP to cyclic AMP. After cyclic AMP has produced the expected change of permeability, cyclic AMP is degraded to a physiologically inactive derivative $5'$-AMP. Its inactivation can be prevented, however, by xanthine derivatives such as theophylline. The possible role of theophylline needs some explanation. A high concentration of theophylline stimulates water movement and sodium transport across the isolated bladder. The concentrations needed to achieve this are, however, such as to have little physiological meaning. Nevertheless, in the context of the hypothesis as presented by Orloff & Handler (1967), theophylline should reproduce the effects of vasopressin only if, in the absence of the hormone, the intra-

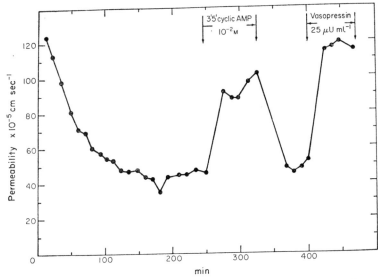

FIG. 8.7. Effect of cyclic 3′,5′-AMP and vasopressin on unidirectional THO permeability of the isolated perfused rabbit
collecting duct. Perfusion solution was isotonic. Note that permeability reached a steady state after 120 min of perfusion (from
Grantham & Burg, 1966).

cellular concentration of cyclic 3′5′-AMP is too small to produce a
physiological response despite its continuous production. The
argument that theophylline can mimic the effects of vasopressin,
and accelerates osmotic water flow in the collecting duct of the
rabbit, remains subject to the criticism of the abnormally high
doses used.

It is of some importance that vasopressin and cyclic AMP have
been shown to have the same effect on net water flow in isolated
collecting ducts of the rabbit (Grantham & Burg, 1966) (Fig. 8.7
and 8.8); that cyclic AMP is present in the urine of normal human
subjects (Butcher & Sutherland, 1962), and that its excretion in
the urine is reduced in patients suffering from diabetes insipidus,
but is increased after administration of vasopressin (Takahashi,
Kaminura, Shinko & Tsuji, 1966). The main support for the
hypothesis comes, however, from the finding that there is a marked
increase in the concentration of the nucleotide in renal tissues and
toad bladder after they have been incubated with vasopressin or

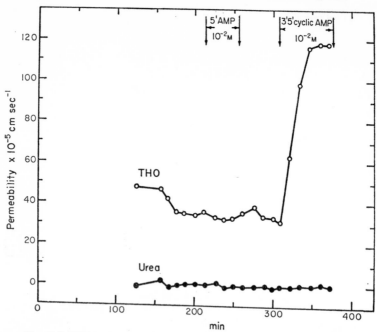

FIG. 8.8. Effect of 5′-AMP and 3′, 5′-AMP on unidirectional THO and urea-^{14}C permeability of collecting tubule. Perfusion solution isotonic (from Grantham & Burg, 1966).

theophylline (Brown, Clarke, Roux & Sherman, 1963; Handler, Butcher, Sutherland & Orloff, 1965). No increase in the concentration of 3′5′-AMP was observed when the same tissues were incubated with insulin or angiotensin. The concentration of nucleotide in control experiments was of the order of 10^{-7} M; when in the presence of either vasopressin or theophylline it increased between twenty- and 100-fold. But even the highest increase of concentration of cyclic adenosine 3′5′-phosphate is far below the concentration of the nucleotide required (10^{-2} M) to elicit a physiologic response.

Bentley (1959, 1960) and Petersen & Edelman (1964) found that an increase of the concentration of calcium in the bathing fluid reduced the hydro-osmotic effect of vasopressin on the isolated toad bladder, but did not modify the effects on sodium transport. Since, however, calcium does not modify the response to exogenous cyclic 3′5′-AMP on either sodium transport or water flow, it has been suggested that cyclic AMP may be formed at two different sites, both sensitive to vasopressin, but one only, that controlling water movement, sensitive to calcium (Orloff & Handler, 1967). The role of calcium in the interpretation of these experiments is critical. Absence of this ion from the fluid bathing the serosal side leads to cell detachment and loss of the function of barrier in the toad bladder. In contrast, elevated levels of calcium (up to 10 mM/l.) in the bathing fluid produce a marked decrease of the sensitivity of the preparation to vasopressin (Bentley, 1959; Schwartz & Walter, 1965), but do not affect either sodium transport or water flux induced by cyclic AMP (Petersen & Edelman, 1964).

How then does the antidiuretic hormone work? There would appear to be little doubt that the hormone has to be bound on a 'receptor' before it can have an effect. The lack of response to vasopressin in the presence of high concentrations of calcium has been interpreted as the result of a competitive antagonism between the ion and the polypeptide for the same receptor. Whether the ensuing hydro-osmotic and natriuretic effects are due to a disulphide–sulphydryl interchange capable of dilating channels for water and sodium or whether the interchange triggers off the stimulation of synthesis of cyclic 3'5'-adenosine phosphate which in turn opens the channels for water and urea and for sodium is still not clear. Both views, however, imply the existence of some kind of pores, the inference being that water goes through the cell membrane. According to Ginetzinsky's hypothesis, however, water would penetrate the tissues through their depolymerized basement membranes and thus move in between cells, a view which would agree with the histological observations of Ganote et al. (1968) on the renal collecting ducts of the rabbit. It might then be possible to visualize the mechanism of action of vasopressin as follows: first, adsorption of the hormone on a 'receptor'; second, a possible disulphide–sulphydryl interchange; third, stimulation of production of cyclic 3'5'-adenosine monophosphate; fourth, apocrine secretion of hyaluronidase. In spite of its attraction such a scheme is subject to criticism since according to most authors hyaluronidase does not mimic the action of either vasopressin or 3'5'-AMP on the isolated frog skin or toad bladder preparation. On the other hand, cyclic 3'5'-adenosine monophosphate is able to mimic the different effects attributed to vasopressin only when abnormally

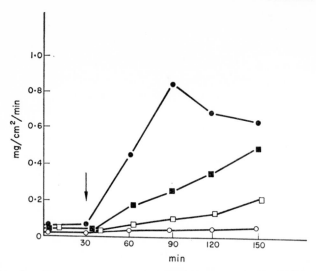

FIG. 8.9. The influence of hyaluronidase and vasopressin on the permeability of frog urinary bladder for water. Ordinate =mg of water transported through the wall of urinary bladder (1 cm²/min). The arrow shows the moment of the addition of hyaluronidase (5 mg/ml.) to the Ringer's solution, pH 5·4 (■—■) or 1 mu./ml. vasopressin to the Ringer's solution, pH 7·6 (●—●). The respective controls are expressed as □—□ and O—O (from Natochin & Shakhmatova, 1968).

large amounts of the substance (10⁻²M) are used, though its highest concentration in tissues is of the order of 10⁻⁸M only. Even if it were correct that the antidiuretic hormone acted by stimulating the synthesis of cyclic 3′5′-AMP, it should be possible to exhaust the action of vasopressin and to reload the toad bladder with ATP, since the amount of ATP available in a tissue is finite. This, however, is not so. Finally, it is still not clear whether cyclic AMP can penetrate the membrane of the collecting ducts (Orloff & Handler, 1964) which may be the reason why when injected intravenously it does not produce an antidiuresis. We are still far from the solution, and shall have to wait until more is known of the physical and chemical changes responsible for what must lead to structural changes in the limiting membranes before the mechanism of action of the antidiuretic hormone is fully understood.

9

RENAL FUNCTION IN THE NEW-BORN MAMMAL

SINCE a foetus may develop, albeit deformed, in spite of the absence of a urinary tract (Windle, 1940; Potter, 1946; Smith, 1951) it has been argued that the kidneys do not function before birth. While Stanier (1960) showed that the mesonephros of foetal rabbits and pigs does not produce any urine, McCance & Stanier (1960) were able to show, however, that the metanephros of rabbit's foetuses (9 days before term) could form a fluid resembling urine. The urea concentration of this fluid was about three-fold that of plasma, while its concentration of chloride was only half that of the blood serum. This suggested that in the metanephros about two thirds of the amount of water filtered by the glomeruli had been reabsorbed and that chloride had been reabsorbed to an even greater extent than water. In 90-day-old pig foetuses, the urine is very dilute. Judging by the degree of concentration of urea and creatinine, little water had been reabsorbed, while in contrast chloride and phosphate appeared to have been reabsorbed very efficiently. In man, it is known that a baby nearly always empties its bladder a few seconds after delivery, even if the latter follows a Caesarean section. The urine must therefore have been formed 'in utero'. The composition of the first urine secreted after birth is not only different from that of the blood serum and of the urine of the mother, but from the urine voided during the first hours *after* birth (McCance & Widdowson, 1953, 1954). The first urine is always markedly hypotonic, it is poor in urea and creatinine, but richer in sodium chloride (McCance & Widdowson, 1954; Dicker, unpublished). On the assumption that the rate of excretion of creatinine represents a measure of glomerular filtration, it might not be unreasonable to conclude that the rate of filtration in the kidney of babies is much smaller before than after birth.

It has been suggested that the composition of the urine formed before birth is that of a fluid elaborated by the kidneys at a time when they were not under the control of the antidiuretic hormone. Though little is known about the release of the antidiuretic hormone in the embryo, neurohypophysial hormones have been shown to exist in the neural lobe of foetuses a long time before birth (Benirsche & McKay, 1953; Dicker & Tyler, 1953). The possibility that the antidiuretic hormone is released in the foetus cannot be ruled out. That immature kidneys can respond to the presence of vasopressin is, however, unlikely (Heller, 1944).

The kidney of the new-born rat resembles that of the foetus of other mammals and man. In contrast to the kidneys of babies, in which the process of nephron formation is complete at birth, in the kidney of the new-born rat most of the Malpighian corpuscules are still in various stages of formation. For instance, according to Kittelson (1917), in the new-born rat there are some 15,000 glomeruli of which more than a third are incompletely formed; two weeks after birth, however, the number of glomeruli has increased to 24,000, with only 30 incompletely developed. In contrast to the rat, in the new-born baby all glomeruli appear to be fully formed (Arataki, 1926). The study of the kidney functions of the new-born rat may therefore throw some light on the renal functions of the human foetus. Bogomolova (1965) studied the cytological and cytochemical changes in the rat's kidney from birth up to old age (30 months). At birth, the rat's kidney is not yet fully formed. The nephrogenic tissue from which the nephrons are formed lies in the peripheral part of the kidney beneath the capsule (Baxter & Yoffey, 1948). The tubular system is not fully formed; the loops of Henle are weakly differentiated, the renal papilla is short and the collecting ducts are few in number. Much of the medullary layer and the papilla consists of interstitial connective tissue (Bogomolova, 1965). Polysaccharides are present in the interstitial tissue. Glycogen inclusions are found in the nephrogenic layer, in the epithelium of the collecting ducts and in the cavity of the papillary ducts and pelvis. In the collecting tubes, the glycogen is localized in the apical part of the cells, from which it is secreted into the lumen of the tube, and hence into the urine. The glycogen secretion ceases when functional differentiation is achieved. No glycogen has been found in the kidneys of adult rats. Its physiological significance in the neonate remains un-explained (Bogomolova, 1965).

In young mice, histological differentiation of the tubular system becomes apparent at about the 15th post-natal day (Longley & Fisher, 1956). According to these authors, in the kidney of the adult mouse, the tubular epithelium of the most proximal segment of the proximal tubule exhibits strong alkaline phosphatase activity, whereas the more distal part of the proximal tubule appears to be devoid of it. In the new-born mouse, however, there is no such differentiation. The differentiation of the two segments of the proximal tubule on the basis of presence of alkaline phosphatase activity develops gradually between the 22nd and the 36th post-natal days. Whether the enzymic activity of the alkaline phos-phatase is related to the reabsorptive capacity of the proximal tubule has not yet been elucidated, though according to Galan (1949) it may be related to the reabsorption of glucose since the maximal tubular reabsorption of glucose in young children (2–11 years old) greatly exceeds that of adults.

Various enzymes have been studied histochemically in the kidneys of new-born rat and the rabbit, which both have at birth an active nephrogenic zone and compared with those of the kidney of guinea-pig, which at birth is fully mature (Wachstein & Bradshaw, 1965). According to these authors there is a lack of enzymic activity in the proximal convoluted tubes of the new-born rat and rabbit. Adult pattern of enzymes was found at about 14th to 16th day after birth in the rat and after 21 to 28 days in the rabbit. New-born guinea-pig kidney lacks glomerular adenosine triphosphatase activity in spite of its otherwise enzymic maturity. In the rat and rabbit kidney no adenosine triphos-phatase can be detected in the tubules. Oxidative enzymes, such as succinic dehydrogenase and acid phosphatase are very active in the renal tubules of the rat and rabbit at birth. Since with the progress of zonal differentiation these enzymes disappear, their presence has been taken as an expression of the immaturity of the kidney. Signs of immaturity can also be seen in the medulla. In the mature kidney, the outer-medulla contains thin descending and thick ascending limbs of the loop of Henle, collecting ducts and capil-laries; whereas the inner medulla consists of both thin descending and ascending limbs of Henle's loops. In the immature kidney of rat or rabbit, however, there is no differentiation between the ascending and descending limbs. Towards the third post-natal week, there appears a slow transformation of the epithelium of the tip of the loop, which becomes thin and translucent with a narrow lumen.

Though parts of the human kidney at birth are not fully developed, all glomeruli seem to have been formed. But according to Peter (1927) though all the glomeruli are formed, the tubules attached to those near the capsule are still very primitive and the loops of Henle are very short. The most central nephrons are in a more advanced stage of development, though they still have many primitive features. In adult life, the glomerular tuft is covered with the thinnest of pavement epithelia. In the human foetus, however, and in the new-born rat, the tuft is covered with a layer of tall columnar cells (Klein, Burdon-Sanderson, Foster & Brunton, 1873; Grünewald & Popper, 1940), which may provide an anatomical basis for the low filtration rates and low clearances observed during early life.

Finally, according to Trueta, Barclay, Daniel, Franklin & Prichard (1947), the renal cortex of the neonatal child makes up a much smaller proportion of the kidney than it does in later life, which suggests that the medullary and juxta-medullary glomeruli may have a particular significance. Trueta et al. (1947) further believe that these glomeruli have a different blood supply from those in the cortex. As stated by McCance (1948) it is possible that the function of these inner nephrons differs from those lying near the cortex and these anatomical differences may underlie the functional differences between the kidneys of the new-born and adult animal. This, however, is only a matter of conjecture.

One of the greatest difficulties in assessing, and hence comparing, renal function at different ages is the choice of parameters used. Whereas, in the adult, it is common usage to express the different functional tests in terms of body weight, or body surface, this, if used for the new-born animal, will give a distorted figure. As suggested by McCance & Widdowson (1953), the best common basis of expression for both new-born and adult animals may be the total water content of their body. The body water of an adult man weighing 70 kg has been estimated to be 42·1 litres. According to Widdowson & Spray (1951) the body water of a baby weighing 2·5 kg is 1·9 l., that of an infant of 3 kg is 2·2 l., and that weighing 3·5 kg is 2·4 l. The kidneys, however, by necessity, will have to handle these greatly different amounts of water.

The average amount of urine excreted by babies during their first day of life is of the order of 14 ml./l. body water; whereas an adult receiving, like the baby, no food and only small amounts of water will excrete during the same period some 17 ml./l. body water. According to McCance & Widdowson (1954) the average total osmolar concentration of the baby's urine during the first 24 hours is of the order of 420 m-osmole/l. The calculated osmolar clearance, therefore, would be 19·6 m-osmole/l. body water/24 hours. In similar circumstances, the estimated osmolar clearance in the adult would be at least 90 m-osmole/l. body water. Therefore the calculated free water clearance would be negative, and amount to

for the baby: − 5·6 ml./l. body water/24 hr and
for the adult: − 73 ml./l. body water/24 hr.

Similar calculations would show that immediately after birth the free-water clearance is of the order of − 7·0 ml./l. body water/24 hr. These figures, though approximate, are interesting. On the assumption that in the new-born baby, as in the adult, the glomerular filtrate is essentially iso-osmotic with the plasma, they indicate that the two most important physiological features of the kidneys, i.e. the reabsorption of water and the reabsorption of solutes, exist already before birth. It would appear, therefore, that the events occurring immediately after birth are less likely to be due to any sudden change in the function of the organ than to changes in the work which the kidneys are called upon to do. The real problem then is to what extent do the kidneys of the new-born animal succeed to adjust their function in their effort to maintain the constancy of the 'milieu interieur'?

Since it would appear that in most mammals *before* birth, and in the pig *after* birth (McCance & Stanier, 1960) the kidneys excrete a urine more dilute than the plasma, the question is whether the new-born animal can respond to an increased water load in a way similar to that of the adult? After receiving 4·5% or 5% of its body weight of water by stomach tube, the rate of urine flow of the new-born rat remains the same as before (Fig. 9.2) (McCance & Wilkinson, 1947; Heller, 1947a, b; Dicker, 1952). This could be attributed partly to a lack of water absorption from the alimentary canal. Heller (1947b) showed, however, that though the whole of the administered water had been absorbed in about 3 hr, no sign

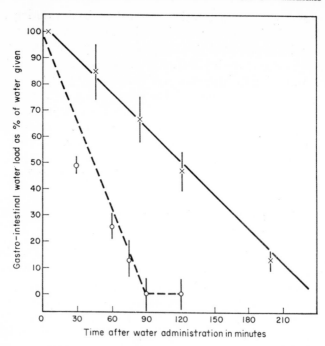

FIG. 9.1. The rate of alimentary water absorption in new-born
(x—x) and in adult (o—o) rats. Both series received 4·5 ml. water/
100 g. The adult rats in addition, received 3 ml. milk/100 g 10 min
before the water was administered. The new-born rats were kept
at 30/31 °C air temperature, the adult rats at 20/21 °C. The slower
rate of water absorption in new-born rats is evident (Heller, 1947).

of water diuresis were observed even after 5 hr. (Fig. 9.1). In
puppies (Adolph, 1943; Dicker, 1952) and infants aged a week or
so (McCance, Naylor & Widdowson, 1954) water administration
is followed by some water diuresis, though it subsided before
50–60% of the water had been excreted. Furthermore, though the
diuresis was accompanied by a decrease in the osmolar concentration of the urine, it never reached the degree of dilution observed
in adult animals (Dicker & Heller, 1951).

The reason for the lack of a renal response to water loading in
the new-born animal remains ill understood. The following considerations may provide a basis for discussion and for further
investigation. In the adult mammal suitably hydrated, there is an

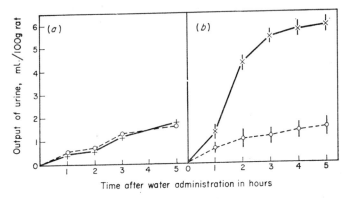

Fig. 9.2. Comparison between the urinary output of new-born and of adult rats after administration of water by the stomach. (a) x—x, mean urinary output of new-born rats after the intragastric injection of 4·5 ml. water/100 g rat; o—o, controls. The figures for the urine volume at various times were obtained by deducting the mean residual urine volume (= mean volume of urine contained in the bladder at the outset of the experiment) from the volume of urine obtained at a given time. (b) x—x, mean urinary output of adult rats which received 3 ml milk/100 g by mouth and 4·5 ml. water/100 g 10 min later (3 ml. milk/100 g rat = approximate content of milk in alimentary tract of new-born rats at outset of diuresis experiments); o—o, mean urinary output of adult rats which received 3 ml. milk/100 g only. The vertical lines indicate the standard error. There is no evidence that the new-born rats excreted any of the administered water during the 5 hours of observation.

Further diuresis experiments on adult rats receiving a preparation of 'full cream dried cows' milk', partly reconstituted to make the concentrations of proteins and fat approximately equal to those of rat milk, gave essentially the same results (Heller, 1947).

increased rate of urine excretion with the accompanying fall in osmolar concentration, which coincides with the absence of anti-diuretic and hyaluronidase activity in the urine. In contrast, the urine of the newly born baby, contains, irrespective of the degree of hydration, appreciable amounts of both antidiuretic and hyaluronidase activity (Dicker & Eggleton, 1960). Since there is good evidence that in the new-born mammal the neurohypophysial hormones may not be bound to the carrier, neurophysin, in the same manner as in the adult (Bargmann, 1949; Dawson, 1953;

Scharrer, 1954; Green & van Bremen, 1955; Rodeck & Caesar, 1956; Rodeck, 1958; Heller & Lederis, 1959; Dicker, 1966) and that the release of these hormones in the neonates does not appear to be controlled in the same way as it is in adults (Dicker, 1966), it might be hypothesized that in the new-born animal the anti-diuretic hormone is continuously released into the blood stream. If this were correct, it would mean that the kidneys of new-born animals, whether hydrated or not, are continuously under the influence of the antidiuretic hormone, though they are not able to respond to it. It would explain also the absence of free-water clearance, and the presence of antidiuretic and hyaluronidase activity in the urine of new-born animals and babies. This inter-pretation, however, is still conjectural and awaits experimental testing.

Be that as it may, the next question is whether the kidneys of new-born mammals can concentrate their urine as adults do. Heller (1949) showed that the specific gravity of urine of new-born rats which had received no food or fluid for 24 hr., was the same

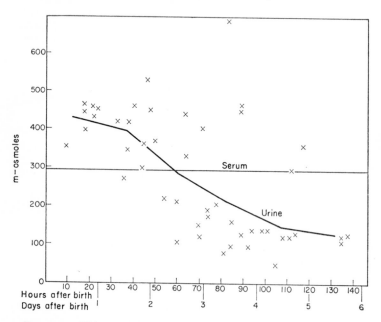

FIG. 9.3. Urinary osmotic pressures (in terms of m-osmolar equivalents) of a series of new-born infants (Heller, 1944).

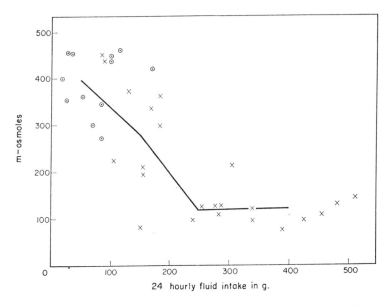

FIG. 9.4. Relation between fluid intake and urinary osmotic pressure (in terms of m-osmolar equivalents) of a series of new-born infants. ⊙, infants aged 8–48 hr; x, infants aged 49–135 hr (Heller, 1944).

as that of control animals and that in contrast to what occurs in the adult, withdrawal of food and water produced a decrease of the urine concentration. Whereas the osmolar concentration of the urine of control new-born rats was estimated at 180 ± 14.6 m-osmole/l., that of dehydrated new-born animals was 132 ± 10.5 m-osmole/l. only. It is possible that this fall in the osmolar concentration of the urine may be explained, partly if not entirely, by a reduction of the glomerular filtration rate. According to Heller (1949), however, the lack of urinary concentration could be attributed to a fault in the neurohypophysial mechanism which regulates urinary concentration in the adult. Heller (1947) listed as possible defects: an insufficient production of the antidiuretic hormone or possibly an insufficient development of osmoreceptors. Since Heller published his results before the role of the loops of Henle as a countercurrent multiplier system had been demonstrated, the possibility of an imperfect functioning of the latter should be added to the list.

It is unlikely that the absence of urine concentration in the neonate can be attributed to an insufficient amount of the antidiuretic hormone. The amount of antidiuretic activity has been estimated

TABLE 9.1

The antidiuretic and oxytocic hormone content of human posterior pituitary glands (means and their standard errors)

	Adults	New-born infants
Wt of anterior lobe (wet, mg.)	435 ±33·8	60 ±5·9
Wt of posterior lobe (wet, mg.)	131 ±6·5	15 ±1·6
Wt of posterior lobe as percentage of whole pituitary gland	24·5 ±1·82	23·6 ±2·22
Wt of posterior lobe (dry, mg.)	19·8 ±1·4	2·4 ±0·2
Solids in posterior lobe (%)	14·9 ±0·53	15·8 ±1·38
Antidiuretic activity:		
(a) (mu./posterior lobe)	14,570 ±1580	375 ±40
(b) (mu./mg. dry posterior lobe tissue)	761 ±58	166 ±25
Oxytocic activity:		
(a) (mu./posterior lobe)	13,850 ±1085	387 ±20
(b) (mu./mg. dry posterior lobe tissue)	747 ±45	150 ±38

(from Heller & Zaïmis, 1949)

in glands of new-born rats (Heller, 1947a), guinea-pigs, kittens and puppies (Dicker & Tyler, 1953), chicks (Dicker, 1967) and new-born infants (Heller & Zaïmis, 1949) (Table 9.1). The amounts present are small when compared with those found in adult animals. Attempts to interpret the results by correlating them to an arbitrarily chosen parameter like body weight or body surface may be misleading. For instance, when referred to body weight the posterior pituitary gland of new-born babies was found to contain about 185 mu./kg, which is not very different from the estimated content in the adult: 224 mu./kg. When, however, these figures were expressed in terms of body surface, the amount of antidiuretic hormone was 17 for the infant and 84 mu./100 cm² in the adult (Heller, 1954). If body water is chosen as a common measure, then these amounts are 150 and 340 mu./l. respectively. But it is not so much the actual amount of hormones that matter. The neurohypophysis acting as a store, the quantity of vasopressin in it represents the difference between the rate at which it is synthesized and that at which it is released. Little, if anything, is known as to the rate at which it is synthesized and transported to the neural lobe. Neural lobes of new-born rats deprived of milk for 24 hr contain about 25% less antidiuretic activity than the pituitaries of litter-mate controls which stayed with their mother (Heller, 1960). Likewise, the ingestion of hypertonic NaCl solution (2·9%) by new-born rats increased the antidiuretic activity content of the urine two-fold from 0·3 to 0·6 mu./100 g (Heller, 1960). These results suggest that the osmoregulatory apparatus in the neonate rat responds to the stimulation of dehydration and that relatively large amounts of antidiuretic hormone are released. They also confirm that in contrast to what has been found in the adult the urine of the fully hydrated new-born animals contains a substantial amount of antidiuretic activity, presumably of neurohypophysial origin.

An assessment of the action of the antidiuretic hormone on the kidney of new-born animals or infants meets with difficulties. It is customary to estimate the response of the mammalian kidney to vasopressin by the inhibitory effect of a given dose of the hormone on a water diuresis. This technique is difficult to apply to the new-born mammal, since it is not possible either to produce a water diuresis or to make it empty its bladder at regular intervals. In an attempt to overcome this, Heller (1944) estimated the concentration rather than the volume of urine. Here is the description of his technique: 'A urine specimen from a new-born child was collected and a given dose of posterior pituitary extract injected intramuscularly. Samples of urine voided spontaneously at the two following occasions were then taken and the freezing point of all specimens determined. In order to compare the effect of the antidiuretic principle on the urine secretion of the new-born child with that on the adult an equivalent amount of posterior pituitary extract was injected into adults who drank 100 ml. water per square metre body surface at intervals of 15 min throughout the duration of the experiment. Urine samples of adults were collected at exactly the same time as those at which the infants had emptied their bladder spontaneously.' The doses of antidiuretic hormone injected in both infant and adults were either 125 mu. or 250 mu./m². In the case of new-born babies, the first urine collected after the injection of vasopressin was slightly more concentrated than the urine obtained before the injection, but the second sample after the injection always showed a return to the pre-injection level.

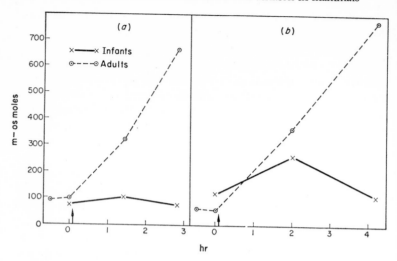

FIG. 9.5. A comparison of the effect of equivalent doses of posterior pituitary extract on the urinary osmotic pressure (in terms of m-osmolar equivalents) of new-born infants and of adults. (a) At the time marked by arrow intramuscular injection of 125 mu./m² into the infant Sh. (5th day of extra-uterine life) and the adult subject Pa. Absolute doses: 25 mu. and 210 mu. respectively. (b) At the time marked by arrow intramusular injection of 250 mu./m² into the infant Ma. (5th day of life) and the adult subject Du. Absolute doses: 50 mu. and 500 mu. respectively (Heller, 1944).

When compared with the effect of similar doses of vasopressin in adults, it was clear that the kidney of the new-born baby was highly insensitive to the antidiuretic hormone (Fig. 9.5). Similar results have been shown in new-born animals. In a recent series of experiments on 5-day-old rats, injected subcutaneously with 200 mu. vasopressin/100 g the concentration of urine collected three hours after the injection averaged 380 m-osmole/l. Though the urine collected must have been a mixture of the urine secreted before and after the injection its osmolar concentration was similar to that of control animals. When repeating the experiments on adult rats, however, the concentration of urine after subcutaneous injection of 200 mu. vasopressin/100 g averaged 950 m-osmole/l. (Dicker & Morris, unpublished). Though these experiments illustrate the marked insensitivity of the kidney of newly born mammals to the antidiuretic hormone, they fail to indicate the reason for it. The first question to be answered is: does vasopressin act on the collecting ducts of new-born mammals in the same way as in the adult?

Since the kidneys of most neonates are immature, it might be that the protein receptor of the target site is not fully receptive yet. Ginsburg & Jayasena (1968) prepared from various organs from adult pigs and guinea-pigs a protein fraction which contained an antigen reacting with antineurophysin serum. The fraction from the kidney bound vasopressin but not oxytocin. Ginsburg & Jayasena suggested that the term 'extra-neurohypophysial neuro-physin' be used tentatively to describe this protein fraction. This fraction shares several binding properties with neurophysin obtained from the neural lobe. Since the neurophysin from the neurohypophysis appears to undergo a process of maturation (Papez, 1940; Bargman, 1949; Auer, 1951; Dawson, 1953; Benirschke & McKay, 1953; Scharrer, 1954; Diepen, Engelhardt & Smith-Agreda, 1954; Green & van Bremen, 1955; Rodeck & Caesar, 1956; Rodeck, 1958; Amoroso, Harrison, Harrison-Matthews, Rowlands, Bourne & Sloper, 1958; Heller & Lederis, 1959; Dicker, 1966; Dicker & King, 1969), a similar process might affect a renal protein fraction which appears to be so similar to the protein-carrier in the neurohypophysis. If this is so, it would be possible to postulate that the hormone is poorly bound in the receptors in the kidney, which in turn would explain its lack of effect.

Another explanation may be the undeveloped countercurrent system in the medulla. All histological investigations of the kidney of the new-born mammal mention the absence or the lack of differentiation of the loop of Henle. Furthermore, in the rat the medulla and the papilla of the new-born animal consists mainly of interstitial connective tissue (Bogomolova, 1965). Little, if anything, is known about the arrangement of vasa recta. In an attempt to see whether a concentration gradient exists in the medulla of kidneys of new born rats and guinea-pigs a technique essentially similar to that described by Opie (1949); Robinson (1950) and Ullrich et al. (1955) was used. Slices from the cortex and the medulla of kidneys from 5-day-old rats were cut on a Stadie & Riggs (1944) microtome. The thickness of the slices was of approximately 0·25 mm. The slices were incubated in a Robinson Ringer solution, buffered at pH 7·3 and oxygenated. Changes in weight of slices were followed at 10-min intervals for a period of up to 1 hr. In control experiments, slices from both the cortex and the medulla were in osmotic equilibrium in solutions of 300 m-osmole/l. When the new-born rats had been injected with vasopressin (20 mu./100 g body weight) or had been given 5 ml./100 g of 1·8% NcCl by stomach tube, slices from the medulla were found to be in osmotic equilibrium with solutions of an osmolarity equal, or nearly equal, to that of the urine. The highest osmolar concentration of urine observed in these experiments was of the order of 400 m-osmole, and the highest osmolar concentration of the incubation fluid in which slices from the medulla were in osmotic equilibrium was 380–400 m-osmole/l. The highest concentration achieved by the kidneys of these new-born rats was equivalent to less than 1·2% NaCl solution. In adult rats injected with an equivalent dose of 20 mu. vasopressin/ 100 g, the osmolar concentration near the lower third of the

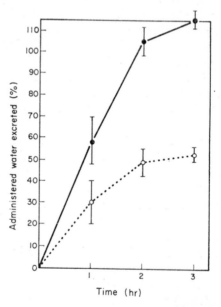

FIG. 9.6. Comparison between the urinary output of adult and new-born guinea-pigs after administration of 5 ml. water/100 g body weight. ●—●, mean urinary output of adult animals; o—o, mean urinary output of new-born animals. The vertical lines indicate the standard error (Dicker & Heller, 1951).

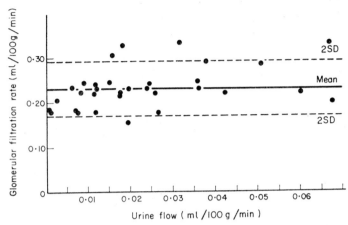

FIG. 9.7. Relation between inulin clearance (=glomerular filtration rate) and rate of urine flow in adult guinea-pigs (Dicker & Heller, 1951).

medulla and that of the urine was of the order of 1300 m-osmole/l., equivalent to 4·0% NaCl solution (Dicker & Morris, unpublished). Similar experiments performed on new-born guinea-pigs (12–18 hr

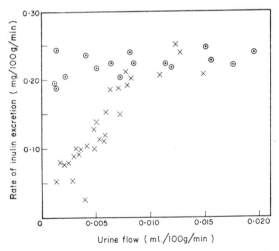

FIG. 9.8. Relation between rate of inulin excretion and rate of urine flow in new-born and adult guinea-pigs. x, new-born animals; ⊙, adult animals (Dicker & Heller, 1951).

old) indicated the existence in the renal medulla of a concentration gradient similar to that observed in the adult (Dicker & Morris, unpublished). This is not surprising since guinea-pigs are born almost adult: for instance they show co-ordinated locomotion and position reflexes, they are not blind, their incisors and molars are present and their tissue metabolism is very much the same as that of adult guinea-pigs. As for their renal function, the new-born guinea-pig excretes a smaller fraction of a standard dose of administered water in a given time than adults, though the ability of the new-born guinea-pig to concentrate its urine was similar to that of the adult animal (Figs. 9.6, 9.7 and 9.8) (Dicker & Heller, 1951).

These observations confirm indirectly the role of the loops of Henle, since in its absence little urinary concentration can be achieved. They do not exclude, however, the possibility that the collecting ducts of the neonate rat may be less sensitive to vasopressin than those of the adult animal. Too little of the renal physiology of the neonate is known to be able to draw conclusions which are more than tentative. To this day there has been only one attempt to use micropuncture technique in the new-born animal (Stanier, 1969). Until more is known on the subject, the only valid conclusion seems to be that the absence or lack of efficiency of loops of Henle functioning as a countercurrent multiplier system is responsible for the poor ability of the kidneys of new-born animals to concentrate their urine.

10

DISCUSSION, SPECULATIONS, CONCLUSION

'The normal is gone because it never was'.
'Plato and Clementine'
H. W. Smith, 1947

IT is time to see whether the many observations reported so far can be welded so as to explain how the kidneys produce urine which can be either more dilute or more concentrated than the plasma.

In kidneys of all vertebrates with the exception of those of some teleost fishes, the formation of urine starts with the separation from the plasma of an iso-osmotic ultrafiltrate. All vertebrates can secrete a urine more dilute than the initial ultrafiltrate, but only some can produce a urine more concentrated than their plasma. All vertebrates, besides having kidneys, have some kind of anti-diuretic hormone. Though it is not yet clear what the functions of antidiuretic hormones are in primitive animals such as the cartilagenous or bony fishes, in other vertebrates, from amphibians to mammals, their function appears to be essentially that of increasing the permeability to water of certain membranes otherwise relatively impermeable to it. If the cells of such a membrane are bathed by two solutions of different osmotic pressure, the effect of the polypeptide on the membrane tends to lead to the establishment of an osmotic equilibrium between the two solutions. Thus in amphibians arginine–vasotocin, by increasing the permeability of renal collecting ducts or of the bladder, will allow water from a hypo-osmotic urine to pass through their membranes until equilibrium has been reached; and since the osmotic pressure in the kidneys or anywhere else in the body of the frog is never above that of its plasma, this will be the maximum osmotic pressure of urine. In higher vertebrates, however, the renal medulla may have an osmotic pressure several times that of the plasma. In these animals,

149

vasopressin will act in the same way as vasotocin in amphibians, and the highest osmolar concentration of the urine will be that existing in the tip of the medulla.

The problem faced by lower vertebrates such as amphibians which live mostly in water is more that of an excess rather than a lack of water. In this respect the hydrated frog and a water-loaded mammal are in a similar situation: both have to get rid of an excess of water. It may be that the production of a dilute urine is a primitive function of the kidneys.

In contrast with most higher vertebrates, in lower vertebrates glomerular filtration increases with hydration. In all mammals, birds, amphibians and most fishes, the proximal convoluted tubule is endowed with the property of reducing the volume of the glomerular filtrate by an amount which is proportionately very much the same, and the highest rate of urine flow does not exceed, therefore, the amount of filtrate left over after the major portion of it has been reabsorbed. This is confirmed by the observation that the highest rate of urine flow in lower and higher vertebrates approximates to 20% of the rate of glomerular filtration, such rates being observed only in the absence of anti-diuretic hormones. But since the reabsorption along the proximal convoluted tubule is an iso-osmotic process, it cannot account for the fact that the urine may be up to twenty times or so more diluted than the plasma. In theory this could be achieved by secretion of water into the lumen of the distal part of the nephron. Quite apart from other objections, such a process would lead to a rate of urine flow which may be in excess of what is available after the reduction of the filtrate has taken place in the proximal con-voluted tubules. If, as it would appear, there is an upper limit to the rate of urine excretion, its ultimate dilution must result from the reabsorption of osmotically active material, particularly sodium and chloride ions. Since active reabsorption of sodium has been shown to operate all along the renal tubule of lower and higher vertebrates and is fairly independent of the rate of urine flow, it will account for the production of a urine of low osmotic pressure and explain why normally hydrated frogs produce an abundant and dilute urine. When an amphibian needs to conserve water, its anti-diuretic hormone will be released in the blood. As the hormone reaches the kidney, it will alter the permeability of its collecting ducts and water will pass along the osmotic gradient existing between the hypo-osmotic liquid in the lumen and the rest of the kidney. This passive reabsorption of water will continue until osmotic equilibrium is achieved, and will lead to a reduction of urine flow.

In mammals, dilution of urine is effected broadly in the same way as in lower vertebrates by the reabsorption of sodium especially in the distal parts of the nephrons. Any substance which impairs the normal transport of sodium produces an increase of the osmolar concentration of the urine without necessarily influencing the rate of urine secretion. This is roughly the way in which most diuretic drugs act.

This schematic representation of how dilution of urine is achieved by the kidneys of vertebrates, does not take into account the peculiar anatomy of nephrons in mammals. It seems almost as if there was an 'internal contradiction' in the physiology of the kidney since it can produce a very dilute urine in the presence of a countercurrent system whose function is clearly that of concentration. When 30 to 50 ml. water per kg body weight is given by stomach tube to a rat, dog or man, the onset of diuresis follows water absorption with a time lag, during which dilution and ultimately disappearance of the antidiuretic hormone from the blood is achieved. When vasopressin has completely disappeared from the bloodstream the distal portion of the nephron is practically impermeable to water. Thus, in theory, the existence of an osmotic gradient in the medulla is irrelevant to the mechanism of dilution of urine. However, experiments show that this is not so. According to Ullrich et al. (1955) 35 min after the administration to a dog of 50 ml. water per kg by stomach tube, the osmolar concentration of the inner medulla of the kidney fell from some 2400 to 500 m-osmole/l. What is it that allows the osmotic gradient to disappear? The efficiency of the renal countercurrent system depends inter alia on the number and the length of the loops of Henle in the inner medulla, the rate at which sodium is 'pumped', the velocity of the fluid that moves through the system and the rate of blood flow through the vasa recta. A change in any of these may affect the efficiency of the system. Furthermore, though these factors are essential for the production of a high concentration of solutes towards the tip of the papilla, the problem of its maintenance is still not quite clearly understood. In 1958 Berliner et al. suggested that it could be explained by postulating the existence

F

of mechanisms by which water is shunted across the tops of the vasa recta, and this might prevent sodium and urea being washed out from the medulla into the arcuate veins. This interpretation awaits confirmation.

In higher mammals, water diuresis is not accompanied by an increased renal blood flow. This, however, does not mean that it is not accompanied by a redistribution of the blood flow in the kidney. In 1947 Trueta et al. reported that stimulation of renal nerves shunted blood from the renal cortex to the medulla. These experiments which at the time provoked an enormous controversy, have been confirmed recently by Pomeranz, Birtch and Barger (1968) who were able to demonstrate that a mild stimulation of the renal nerves reflexly through the carotid sinus or directly by stimulation of the splanchnic nerve or the denervation of baro receptors produce a decrease of flow in the outer cortical peritubular capillaries accompanied by an increase of blood flow through the outer medulla, without affecting the total renal blood flow. More evidence of redistribution of glomerular filtration has come from Horster & Thurau (1968) who showed that the total amount of fluid filtered through the glomeruli of a kidney does not come from a homogeneous population of glomeruli. This agrees with ana-tomical and histological findings which have shown that according to their size (Adebahr, 1962; Munkacsi & Palkovits, 1965), the structure of their vascular pole (Edwards, 1956; Faarup, 1965; Ljungquist, 1964; Moffat, 1967) and the number of long loops of Henle (Lechene, Corby & Morel, 1966; Sperber, 1944) glomeruli can be divided into two distinct groups: the superficial and the juxta-medullary glomeruli. Horster & Thurau (1968) demon-strated further that in rats, out of a total of 30,000 glomeruli per kidney, 6733 nephrons are of the juxta-medullary and 23,267 of the superficial type. Though the amount of filtrate formed varies according to the type of glomeruli, all glomeruli within a cortical layer produce filtrates of a similar order of magnitude. Their respective contribution to the total filtrate, however, can vary. For instance, in rats fed on a low sodium diet (daily intake 0·74 m-equiv NaCl) with a total glomerular filtration rate of 0·94±0·16 ml./min/g kidney, 22·4% of it comes from the juxta-medullary glomeruli, and the remaining 77·6% from the others. In rats fed on a high salt diet (daily intake 10–12 m-equiv NaCl), the total glomerular filtration increased from 0·94 to 1·01 ±

0·24 ml./min, i.e. by 7·4%, but this increase was not equally distributed among the two types of glomeruli. Whereas the filtration rate of single superficial glomeruli increased by 62%, from $23·5 \pm 6·4$ to $38·1 \pm 11·3 \times 10^{-6}$ ml./min/g kidney, that of single juxta-medullary glomeruli decreased by 71·5% from $58·2 \pm 13·6$ to $16·5 \pm 6·6 \times 10^{-6}$ ml./min/g kidney.

It would be tempting to speculate that intrarenal distribution of single nephron filtration may vary, even when the total glomerular filtration remains unchanged, as during water diuresis. In this hypothesis a lack of vasopressin, the dilution of plasma or the stimulation of volume receptors following water loading, would alter the distribution of blood to the medulla or produce an increase of the filtration rate of cortical glomeruli at the expense of juxta-medullary nephrons, or a combination of both. Since cortical nephrons have short loops of Henle this, together with an increase of flow through the vasa recta, would contribute to the reduction of the osmotic gradient in the medulla and eventually to its dissipation. Recently, it has been shown that in rats suffering from hereditary hypothalamic diabetes insipidus the filtration rate of the deep nephrons was low, but it could be increased by administration of antidiuretic hormone. These findings support strongly the suggestion that an increase of filtration rate of the juxta-medullary glomeruli leads to an increase of the amount of solutes delivered into the countercurrent system (Horster, Schnermann & Thurau, 1969; Schnermann, 1969).

Nephrons with either long or short loops of Henle exist in rats. In the dog, however, according to Sperber (1944) all nephrons have long loops. If this is correct, a redistribution of blood between cortical and juxta-medullary glomeruli could not account for the dissipation of the osmotic gradient in the renal medulla of this animal. But Sperber's observation was made on one dog only and preliminary studies with silastic injections of tubules made by Pomeranz et al. (1968) suggest that the nephrons in the outer cortex of the kidney of dogs do have short loops while those in the inner cortex have long loops of Henle. If it could be demonstrated that the anatomy of the kidney of the dog is really similar to that of other animals (Peter, 1909) which have a water diuresis, this might explain why certain rodents such as Meriones or Gerbil, which have nephrons with long loops only, are unable to excrete

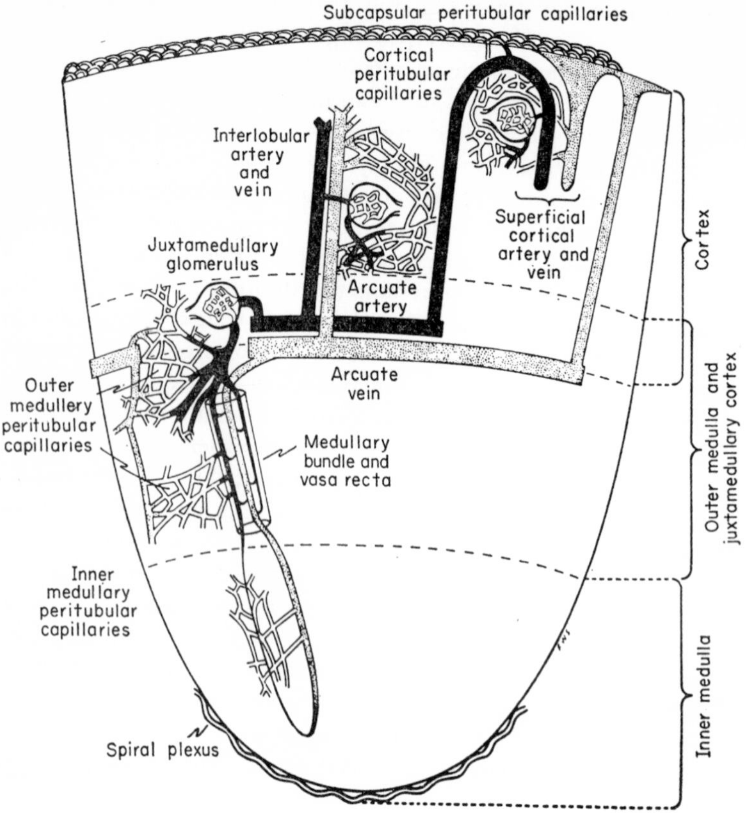

FIG. 10.1. Diagram of the vascular architecture of the normal kidney of a dog. The drawing was made from a series of silicone rubber microvascular casts (see Pomeranz *et al.*, 1968).

extra water given by stomach tube (see chap. 2) and hence to have a water diuresis.

Be that as it may, how does a mammal, while in water diuresis, and therefore without an osmotic gradient in the medulla of its kidney, respond to the release or the injection of a small amount of vasopressin? Though at the time of the administration of the antidiuretic hormone the osmotic pressure of the medulla may not be appreciably different from that of the renal cortex, it will be markedly higher than that of the very dilute urine in the lumen of the collecting ducts. There is thus an osmotic gradient between the inside and the outside of the ducts. A slight increase of permeability of the wall of the ducts to water, as produced by the smallest effective dose of vasopressin, will lead to water leaving the urine and hence produce an antidiuretic effect. Assuming that the hormone remains effective, the antidiuresis will last until osmotic equilibrium has been reached. That this is the most likely explanation of the onset of an antidiuretic response can be derived from the observation that no amounts of vasopressin are able to reduce the urine flow and produce an increase of its osmolar concentration when administered to animals either in osmotic diuresis or while they are dehydrated. In neither case is there an appreciable difference between the osmotic pressure of the urine in the collecting ducts and in the medulla, and therefore an increase of the permeability to water of the wall of the ducts cannot have an effect. Though diffusion of water may take place, it is only when a gradient of hydrostatic or osmotic pressure exists that a transfer of water will occur. This also explains why the injection of vasopressin during water diuresis never results in the secretion of a urine as concentrated as that produced during dehydration: in either case, the concentration of the urine cannot exceed that in the renal medulla.

Towards the end of a water diuresis, there must be reconstitution of the osmotic gradient in the medulla, but how this is achieved is not known. It is tempting to speculate that it is due to the reverse process that has been postulated for its dissipation, i.e. that a redistribution of flow through the nephrons in favour of juxta-medullary nephrons with long loops of Henle takes place. To be effective this process should then be accompanied by a reduction of flow through the vasa recta and a shunting of water across the top of the vasa recta into the arcuate veins, as suggested by Berliner et al. (1958). It is difficult to see how this complicated reorganization of the medulla can be achieved without nervous and/or hormonal control. Evidence for either is still lacking though some recent experiments point to their possible existence. For instance, intra-arterial injections of noradrenaline have been shown to produce a dilatation of vessels in the outer medulla, which can be reversed by adrenergic blocking drugs such as phenoxybenzamine (Pomeranz et al., 1968). Though no adrenergic nerve fibres have been found in the renal medulla of the rat or the rabbit (Nilson, 1965; Moffat, 1967), according to McKenna & Angelakos (1968) there are some adrenergic nerve terminals associated with vasa recta in the kidney of the dog. On the other hand Fourman (1966) found in the thick ascending limb of the loop of Henle of rats cholinesterase activity which increased with dehydration. Since this enzyme has been found in that part of the loop which is responsible for the active transport of sodium out of the ascending limb, it is conceivable that cholinesterase activity is linked with sodium transport and may, therefore, be involved in the reconstitution and maintenance of the osmotic gradient. Another hypothesis is that the sodium 'pump' in the ascending limb of the loop of Henle may be 'reactivated' by cyclic 3′5′-AMP. Since it has been suggested that the action of vasopressin is mediated through that of cyclic 3′,5′-adenosine monophosphate, it might be possible that vasopressin, besides acting on the permeability of cells to water, may act also, though indirectly, on sodium transport. Clearly there is great scope for further investigation.

It remains to be examined whether the anatomy of the loops of Henle and their attendant vasculature in the medulla is really appropriate for the existence of an effective countercurrent system. The models suggested and discussed by Hargitay & Kuhn (1951), Kuhn & Ramel (1959), Thurau et al. (1962), Pinter & Shohet (1963) and others (see chap. 5) have been criticized by Stephenson (1966) on the ground that none of them made provision in their analysis for energy required to perform work at the site of solute transport. Though this may represent an obvious weakness in the mathematical analysis, evidence provided by micropuncture techniques has been able to satisfy nearly all criticisms, especially since Jamison et al. (1957) were able to show that the osmolality of the fluids taken from descending and ascending limbs were markedly different, the osmolality of the fluid in the ascending limb being more dilute than that in the descending limb by some 117 m-osmole/l.

So much of the interpretation of the countercurrent system rests on the evidence provided by micropuncture techniques of nephrons that one cannot help wondering whether the results obtained really represent what happens in the kidney of a non-anaesthetized mammal. Horster & Thurau (1968) have tried to answer some of the most obvious objections which have worried researchers engaged in these investigations. Since according to them the validity of many data 'depends critically on the assumption that intratubular flow dynamics proximal to the site of micropuncture are not affected by the quantitative collection of the tubular fluid at the puncture site', they performed carefully controlled experiments from which they concluded, first that the velocity of flow in the punctured proximal convolutions was the same as that of adjacent non-punctured tubules; second, that the luminal diameter of the tubular segment proximal to the site of puncture was the same during the puncture as during the period preceding it, and the same was true for punctured loops of Henle. Third, the exposure of the renal papilla which is necessary in many of these experiments did not affect the dynamics of flow in the long loops of Henle. Fourth, re-collections of tubular fluid in the same tubular segment demonstrated the reproducibility of the results. It must be remembered, however, that no micropuncture of any parts of nephrons has been achieved during the course of a water diuresis and that the ability of the kidney to concentrate the urine is impaired as a result of puncturing nephrons.

Even though the role of the descending and ascending limbs of the loops of Henle as a countercurrent multiplier system has been well established, the problem of the maintenance of the osmotic gradient, i.e. the mechanism which prevents sodium and urea from being washed out from the medulla into the arcuate veins, is far from being solved. To be effective, the countercurrent exchange requires that the descending and ascending vessels of the vasa recta run parallel to each other for a sufficient distance to allow enough time for diffusion to take place. The circulation in the inner medulla satisfies these conditions; but the anatomy of the capillaries in the outer medulla does not appear to be appropriate for an effective countercurrent exchange since a large fraction of the blood drained by these capillaries bypasses the vasa recta and enters the arcuate vein directly (Moffat & Fourman, 1963; Pomeranz et al., 1968). In addition, the part of the venous return which enters the vasa recta in the outer medulla joins these vessels very close to the arcuate vein so that the distance during which blood can be submitted to the action of a countercurrent exchanger system is far too short. The validity of these criticisms is supported by the results of estimation of the concentration of proteins in the descending vessels of the vasa recta which show that there is practically no increase of their concentration in the outer medulla (Wilde & Vorburger, 1967).

Without doubt more work is required. Observations that have led step by step to the understanding of the role of the loops of Henle remain among the most arresting and stimulating contributions towards the elucidation of the mechanism of urine concentration and dilution in mammals. But as Claude Bernard (1865) said, 'Les idées et les théories de nos prédécesseurs ne doivent être conservées qu'autant qu'elles représentent l'état de la science, mais elles sont évidemment destinées à changer, à moins que l'on admette que la science ne doive plus faire de progrès, ce qui est impossible.'

REFERENCES

'Credo ut Intellegam'
St Augustine

Abramow, M., Burg, M. B. & Orloff, J. (1967). Chloride flux in rabbit kidney tubules *in vitro*. *Am. J. Physiol.* **213**, 1249–1253.

Adebahr, G. (1962). Beitrag zur Morphologie der vasa afferentia und efferentia der juxtamedullären Glomeruli der Menschlichen Niere. *Z. mikrosk. anat. Forsch.* **68**, 48–62.

Adolph, E. F. (1943). *Physiological Regulations*. Lancaster, Pa: Cattell Press.

Ahmed, A. B. J., George, B. C., Gonzalez-Auvert, C. & Dingman, J. F. (1967). Increased plasma arginine–vasopressin in clinical adreno-cortical insufficiency and its inhibition by glucosteroids. *J. clin. Invest.* **46**, 111–117.

Amoroso, E. C., Harrison, R. J., Harrison-Matthews, L., Rowlands, I. W., Bourne, G. H. & Sloper, J. C. (1958). Hypothalamo-neuro-hypophysial neurosecretion. *Int. Rev. Cytol.* **7**, 337–389.

Andersen, B. & Ussing, H. H. (1957). Solvent drag on non-electrolytes during osmotic flow through isolated toad skin and its response to antidiuretic hormone. *Acta physiol. scand.* **39**, 228–239.

Appelboom, J. W., Brodsky, W. A., Tuttle, W. S. & Diamond, I. (1958). The freezing point depression of mammalian tissues after sudden heating in boiling distilled water. *J. gen. Physiol.* **41**, 1153–1169.

Arataki, M. (1926). On the postnatal growth of the kidney, with special reference to the number and size of the glomeruli (Albino rat). *Am. J. Physiol.* **36**, 399–436.

Aroskar, J. P., Chan, W. Y., Stouffer, J. E., Schneider, C. H., Murti, V. V. S. & Du Vigneaud, V. (1964). Renal excretion and tissue distribution of radioactivity after administration of tritium-labelled oxytocin to rats. *Endocrinology.* **74**, 226–232.

Auer, J. (1951). Postnatal cell differentiation in the hypothalamus of the hamster. *J. comp. Neurol.* **95**, 17–41.

Aukland, K. & Krog, J. (1960a). Polarographic determination of renal oxygen tension. *Acta physiol. scand.* **50**, suppl. 175, 13–14.

— (1960b). Renal oxygen tension. *Nature, Lond.* **184**, 671–672.

Babics, A. & Rényi-Vamos, F. (1967). Special anatomy of the lymphatic system, in *Lymphatics and Lymph circulation*. New York: Pergamon.

Baer, J. E., Jones, C. B., Spitzer, A. S. & Russo, H. F. (1967). The potassium-sparing and natriuretic activity of N-amidino-3,5-diamino-6-chloropyrazinecarboxamide hydrochloride (amiloride hydrochloride). *J. pharmac. exp. Ther.* **157**, 472–485.

Bainbridge, F. A. & Evans, C. L. (1914). The heart, lung, kidney preparation. *J. Physiol.* **48**, 278–286.

Barger, A. C. (1966). Renal hemodynamic factors in congestive heart failure in 'The physiology of diuretic agents'. *Ann. N.Y. Acad. Sci.* **139**, 273–284.

Bargeton, D., Durand, J., Mensch-Duchêne, J. & Decaud, J. (1958). Echanges de chaleur de la main. *J. Physiol.*, Paris. **50**, 148–160.

Bargmann, W. (1949). Uber die neurosekretorische Verknüpfung von Hypothalamus und Neurohypophyse. *Z. Zellforsch. mikrosk. Anat.* **34**, 610–634.

Baxter, J. S. & Yoffey, J. M. (1948). The postnatal development of renal tubules in the rat. *J. Anat.* **82**, 189–197.

Bayliss, L. E. (1959). *Principles of General Physiology*, vol. 1, The physico-chemical background. London: Longmans.

— (1960). *Principles of General Physiology*, vol. 2, General physiology. London: Longmans.

— (1966). *Living Control Systems*. London: The English Universities Press.

Bayliss, L. E., Kerridge, P. M. T. & Russell, D. S. (1933). The excretion of protein by the mammalian kidney. *J. Physiol.* **77**, 386–398.

Bayliss, L. E. & Walker, A. M. (1930). The electrical conductivity of glomerular urine from the frog and from *Necturus*. *J. biol. Chem.* **87**, 523–540.

Bazett, H. C., Love, L., Newton, M., Eisenberg, L., Day, R. & Forster, R. (1948). Temperature changes in blood flowing in arteries and veins in man. *F. appl. Physiol.* **1**, 3–19.

Bell, G. H., Davidson, J. N. & Scarborough, H. (1968). *Textbook of Physiology and Biochemistry*. London: Livingstone.

Benirschke, K. & McKay, D. B. (1953). The antidiuretic hormone in foetus and infant. *J. Obst. Gynec.* **1**, 638–649.

Bennett, C. M., Clapp, J. R. & Berliner, R. W. (1967). Micropuncture study of the proximal and distal tubule in the dog. *Am. J. Physiol.* **213**, 1254–1262.

Bentley, P. J. (1959). The effects of ionic changes on water transfer across the isolated urinary bladder of the toad, *Bufo marinus*. *J. Endocr.* **18**, 327–333.

— (1960). The effect of vasopressin on the short-circuit current across the wall of the isolated bladder of the toad, *Bufo marinus*. *J. Endocr.* **21**, 161–170.

— (1962). Hyaluronidase, corticosteroids and the action of neurohypophysial hormones on the urinary bladder of the frog. *J. Endocr.* **24**, 407–413.

— (1965). Hyperglycemic effect of vasotocin in toads. *Nature, Lond.* **206**, 1053–1054.

Bentley, P. J. (1966). The physiology of the urinary bladder of amphibia. *Biol. Rev.* **41**, 275–316.

— (1968*a*). Amiloride: a potent inhibitor of sodium transport across the toad bladder. *J. Physiol.* **195**, 317–330.

— (1968*b*). Action of amphotericin B on the toad bladder: evidence for sodium transport along two pathways. *J. Physiol.* **196**, 703–711.

Berde, B. (1968). Relationship of structure to activity of neurohypophysial hormones. *Excerpta Medica Int. congr.* **161**, 222–223.

Berde, B. & Boissonnas, R. A. (1968). Neurohypophysial hormones and similar polypeptides. Ed. Berde, B., in *Handbuch der Experimentelle Pharmakologie*. Vol. **23**. Berlin: Springer.

Bergen, S. S., Sullivan, R., Hilton, J. G., Willis, S. W. & Van Itallie, T. B. (1960). Glycogenolytic effect of vasopressin in the canine liver. *Am. J. Physiol.* **199**, 136–138.

Berliner, R. W. (1961). Renal mechanisms for potassium excretion. *Harvey Lect.* **55**, 141–171.

Berliner, R. W. & Davidson, D. G. (1957). Production of hypertonic urine in the absence of pituitary antidiuretic hormone. *J. clin. Invest.* **36**, 1416–1427.

Berliner, R. W., Levinsky, N. G., Davidson, D. G. & Eden, M. (1958). Dilution and concentration of the urine and the action of the antidiuretic hormone. *Am. J. Med.* **24**, 730–744.

Bernard, C. (1865). *Introduction à l'étude de la médecine expérimentale*. Paris: Baillière.

— (1876). *Leçons sur la Chaleur Animale*. Paris: Baillière.

Berridge, M. J. & Gupta, B. L. (1967). Fine structural changes in relation to ion and water transport in the rectal papillae of the blowfly, *Calliphora*. *J. cell Sci.* **2**, 89–95.

Bevelander, G. (1935). A comparative study of the branchial epithelium in fishes, with special reference to extrarenal excretion. *J. Morph.* **57**, 335–345.

Blake, D. A., Davies, H. E. F., Emery, E. W. & Wade, E. G. (1956). Renal handling of radioactive potassium in man. *Clin. Sci.* **15**, 277–282.

Bocanegra, M. & Lauson, H. D. (1961). Ultrafiltrability of endogenous antidiuretic hormone from plasma of dogs. *Am. J. Physiol.* **200**, 486–492.

Bogomolova, N. A. (1965). Age changes in kidney of white rat. *Arkh. Anat. Gistol. Embriol.* **48**, 80–85.

Bollett, A. J. & Bonner, W. M. (1963). The presence of hyaluronidase in various mammalian tissues. *Fedn Proc.* **22**, 297.

Bordley, J., Hendrix, J. P. & Richards, A. N. (1933). Quantitative studies of the composition of glomerular urine—XI. The concentration of creatinine in glomerular urine from frogs, determined by an ultra-microadaptation of the Folin method. *J. biol. Chem.* **101**, 255–267.

Bordley, J. & Richards, A. N. (1933). Quantitative studies of the composition of glomerular urine—VIII. The concentration of uric acid in glomerular urine of snakes and frogs determined by an ultra-microadaptation of Folin's method. *J. biol. Chem.* **101**, 193–221.

Boss, J. M. N., Breddy, P. & Cooper, G. F. (1961). Variable and free mucopolysaccharides in the rat's kidney. *J. Physiol.* **157**, 35–36P.

Bossert, W. H. & Schwartz, W. B. (1967). Relation of pressure and flow to control of sodium reabsorption in the proximal tubule. *Am. J. Physiol.* **213**, 793–802.

Bray, G. A. (1960). Freezing point depression of rat kidney slices during water diuresis and antidiuresis. *Am. J. Physiol.* **199**, 915–918.

Breddy, P., Cooper, G. F. & Boss, J. M. N. (1961). Antidiuretic hormone and renal collecting tubules. *Nature, Lond.* **192**, 76.

Brenner, B. M. & Berliner, R. W. (1969). Relationship between extra-cellular volume and fluid reabsorption by the rat nephron. *Am. J. Physiol.* **217**, 6–12.

Brewer, D. B. (1965). Electronmicroscopy of the kidney. *J. clin. Pathol.* **18**, 500–510.

Brodsky, W. A., Austing, M. E., Moxley, T. L. & Grubbs, T. A. (1953). Composition of excreted solutes in experimental diabetes insipidus. Mechanism of urinary dilution. *Am. J. Physiol.* **174**, 448–454.

Brodsky, W. A., Miley, J. F., Kaim, J. T. & Shah, N. P. (1958). Charac-teristics of acid urine after loading with weak organic acids in dogs. Current concepts on renal mechanisms of acidification in relation to data on CO_2 tension. *Am. J. Physiol.* **193**, 108–122.

Brodsky, W. A. & Rapoport, S. (1951). Mechanism of polyuria of diabetes insipidus in man: the effect of osmotic loading. *J. clin. Invest.* **30**, 282–291.

Brodsky, W. A., Rehm, W. S., Dennis, W. H. & Miller, D. G. (1955). Thermodynamic analysis of the intracellular osmotic gradient hypothesis of active water transport. *Science, N.Y.* **121**, 302–303.

Brown, E., Clarke, D. L., Roux, V. & Sherman, G. H. (1963). The stimulation of adenosine $3',5'$-monophosphate production by anti-diuretic factors. *J. biol. Chem.* **238**, 852P.

Brunner, P., Rector, F. C. & Seldin, W. (1966). Mechanism of glomerulo-tubular balance—II. Regulation of proximal tubular reabsorption by volume, as studied by stopped-flow microperfusion. *J. clin. Invest.* **43**, 603–611.

Bull, G. M. (1956). Osmotic diuresis in acute tubular necrosis, in *'Modern Views on the Secretion of Urine'*, ed. WINTON, F. R. London: Churchill.

Burg, M. B., Isaacson, L., Grantham, J. J. & Orloff, J. (1968). Electrical properties of isolated perfused rabbit renal tubules. *Am. J. Physiol.* **215**, 788–794.

Burgess, W. W., Harvey, A. M. & Marshall, E. K. (1933). The site of the antidiuretic action of pituitary extract. *J. Pharmac. exp. Ther.* **49**, 237–249.

Burns, T. W. (1956). Endocrine factors in the water metabolism of the desert mammal, *G. gerbillus*. *Endocrinology* **58**, 243–254.

Butcher, R. W. & Sutherland, E. W. (1962). Adenosine 3′,5′-phosphate in biological materials. *J. biol. Chem.* **237**, 1244–1250.

Cafruny, E. J., Carhart, E. & Farah, A. (1957). Effects of hypophysectomy and hormones on sulphydryl concentrations in rat kidney cells. *Endocrinology* **61**, 143–147.

Capek, C., Rumrich, G. & Ullrich, K. J. (1965). Permeabilität der corticalen Tubulusabschnitte von Ratten für Harnstoff. *Pflügers Arch. ges. Physiol.* **283**, R24.

Chinard, F. P. & Enns, T. (1955). Relative renal excretion patterns of sodium ion, chloride ion, urea, water and glomerular substances. *Am. J. Physiol.* **182**, 247–250.

Civan, M. M., Kedem, O. & Leaf, A. (1966). Effect of vasopressin on toad bladder under conditions of zero net sodium transport. *Am. J. Physiol.* **211**, 569–575.

Clapp, J. R. (1966). Renal tubular reabsorption of urea in normal and protein depleted rats. *Am. J. Physiol.* **210**, 1304–1308.

Clapp, J. R., Rector, F. C. & Seldin, D. (1962). Effect of unreabsorbed anions on proximal and distal transtubular potentials in rats. *Am. J. Physiol.* **202**, 781–786.

Clapp, J. R. & Robinson, R. R. (1966). Osmolality of distal tubular fluid in dog. *J. clin. Invest.* **45**, 1847–1853.

Clapp, J. R., Watson, J. F. & Berliner, R. (1963). Osmolality, bicarbonate concentration and water reabsorption in proximal tubule of the dog nephron. *Am. J. Physiol.* **205**, 273–280.

Cobbin, L. B. & Dicker, S. E. (1962). Some characteristics of plasma and urine hyaluronidase. *J. Physiol.* **163**, 168–174.

Conway, E. J., Fitzgerald, O. & McDougall, T. C. (1946). Potassium accumulation in the proximal convoluted tubules of the frog's kidney. *J. gen. Physiol.* **29**, 305–334.

Cort, J. H. (1963). In 'The mechanism of action of oxytocin and vasopressin and their analogues on the kidney of mammals'. *Proceedings of the 2nd int. Pharmac. Meeting, Prague*, 72–74, vol. 10. Ed. J. Rudinger.

Cortney, M. A., Nagel, W. & Thurau, K. (1966). A micro-puncture study of the relationship between flow rate through the loop of the Henle and sodium concentration in the early distal tubule. *Pflügers Arch. ges. Physiol.* **287**, 286–295.

Crabbe, J. & Nichols, G. (1959). Effects of adrenalectomy and aldosterone on sodium concentration in renal medulla of hydropoenic rats. *Proc. Soc. exp. Biol. Med. N.Y.* **101**, 168–170.

Crabbe, J. & De Weer, P. (1965). Action of aldosterone and vasopressin on the active transport of sodium by the isolated toad bladder. *J. Physiol.* **180**, 560–568.

Crane, M. M. (1927). Observations on the functions of the frog's kidney. *Am. J. Physiol.* **81**, 232–243.

Curran, P. F. & McIntosh, J. R. (1962). A model system for biological water transport. *Nature, Lond.* **193**, 347–348.

Cushny, A. R. (1926). *The Secretion of Urine.* London: Longmans Green.

Cutler, R. E., Kleeman, C. R., Maxwell, M. H. & Dowling, J. T. (1962). Physiologic studies in nephrogenic diabetes insipidus. *J. clin. Endocr. Metab.* **22**, 827–838.

Czaczkes, J. W. & Kleeman, C. R. (1964). The effect of various states of hydration and the plasma concentration on the turnover of anti-diuretic hormone in mammals. *J. clin. Invest.* **43**, 1649–1655.

Dainty, J. & House, C. R. (1966). An examination of the evidence for membrane pores in frog's skin. *J. Physiol.* **185**, 172–184.

Dawson, A. B. (1953). The early appearance of secretion in the neuro-hypophysis and hypothalamic nuclei of the rat. *Anat. Rec.* **117**, 620.

Deetjen, P. & Kramer, K. (1960). Sodium reabsorption and oxygen consumption by the kidneys. *Klin. Wschr.* **38**, 680–682.

Del Greco, F. & De Wardener, H. E. (1956). The effect on urine osmo-larity of a transient reduction in glomerular filtration rate and solute output during a 'water' diuresis. *J. Physiol.* **131**, 307–316.

D'Errico, G. (1907). Uber die physiko-chemischen Verhältnisse und die Harnsekretion bei Hühnern. *Beitr. Z. chem. Physiol. Path.* **9**, 453–460.

De Wardener, H. E. & Del Greco, F. (1955). The influence of solute excretion rate on the production of hypotonic urine in man. *Clin. Sci.* **14**, 715–723.

Diamond, J. M. (1964). The mechanism of isotonic water transport. *J. gen. Physiol* **48**, 15–42.

Diamond, J. M. & Tormey, J. McD. (1966). Role of long extracellular channels in fluid transport across epthelia. *Nature, Lond.* **210**, 817.

Dickens, F. & Weil-Malherbe, H. (1936). Metabolism of normal and tumorous tissue. A note on the metabolism of medulla of kidney. *Biochem. J.* **30**, 659–660.

Dicker, S. E. (1952). Effect of diuretics in newborn rats and puppies. *J. Physiol.* **118**, 384–394.

— (1954). The fate of the antidiuretic activity of pitressin in rats. *J. Physiol.* **124**, 464–475.

— (1957). Urine concentration in the rat during acute and prolonged dehydration. *J. Physiol.* **139**, 108–122.

— (1960). The inactivation of vasopressin and oxytocin *in vitro*. In *Polypeptides which affect Smooth Muscles and Blood Vessels*, pp. 79–82. Ed. SCHACHTER, M. Proc. Symp., London.

— (1963). The mechanism of action of oxytocin and vasopressin and their analogues on the kidneys of mammals from 'Oxytocin, Vaso-pressin and their Structural Analogues'. *Proceedings of the 2nd int. Pharmac. Meeting, Prague.* Ed. RUDINGER, J. vol. 1, 57–74.

— (1966). Release of vasopressin and oxytocin from isolated pituitary glands of adult and newborn rats. *J. Physiol.* **185**, 429–444.

— (1967). Effects of hypertonicity and of high potassium concentration on the rate of release of hormones from neurohypophysial glands of adult and newborn rats and birds, *in vitro*. *J. Physiol.* **192**, 47–48P.

Dicker, S. E. & Eggleton, M. G. (1960). Hyaluronidase and antidiuretic activity in urine of man. *J. Physiol.* **154**, 378–384.

Dicker, S. E. & Eggleton, M. G. (1961). Renal excretion of hyaluronidase and calcium in man during the antidiuretic action of vasopressins and some analogues. *J. Physiol.* **157**, 351–362.

— (1963). Nephrogenic diabetes insipidus. *Clin. Sci.* **24**, 81–89.

— (1964a). The antidiuretic action of hydrochlorothiazide in the hydrated rat. *J. Physiol.* **171**, 377–383.

— (1964b). Renal function in the primitive mammal, *Aplodontia rufa*, with some observations on squirrels. *J. Physiol.* **170**, 186–194.

Dicker, S. E., Eggleton, G. M. & Haslam, J. (1966). The effects of urea and hydrochlorothiazide on the renal functions of rats and domestic fowl. *J. Physiol.* **187**, 247–255.

Dicker, S. E. & Elliott, A. B. (1963). Viscosity reducing activity of tissues in the rat. *J. Physiol.* **165**, 89–97.

— (1967). Water uptake by *Bufo melanostictus* as affected by osmotic gradients, vasopressin and temperature. *J. Physiol.* **190**, 359–370.

Dicker, S. E. & Franklin, C. S. (1966). The isolation of hyaluronic acid and chondroitin sulphate from kidneys and their reaction with urinary hyaluronidase. *J. Physiol.* **186**, 110–120.

Dicker, S. E. & Greenbaum, A. L. (1956). Inactivation of the antidiuretic activity of vasopressin by tissue homogenates. *J. Physiol.* **132**, 199–212.

— (1958). The destruction of the antidiuretic activity of vasopressin by —SH active compounds. *J. Physiol.* **141**, 107–116.

Dicker, S. E. & Haslam, J. (1966). Water diuresis in the domestic fowl. *J. Physiol.* **183**, 225–235.

Dicker, S. E. & Heller, H. (1951). The mechanism of water diuresis in adult and newborn guinea pigs. *J. Physiol.* **112**, 149–155.

Dicker, S. E. & King, V. M. (1969). The preparation, purification and characterization of porcine neurophysin. *J. Physiol.* **202**, 103–104P.

Dicker, S. E. & Morris, C. A. (1969). Unpublished.

Dicker, S. E. & Nunn, J. (1957). Fate and excretion of the pressor activity of vasopressin in rats. *J. Physiol.* **138**, 11–18.

Dicker, S. E. & Tyler, C. (1953). Vasopressor and oxytocic activities of the pituitary glands of rats, guinea-pigs and cats and of human foetuses. *J. Physiol.* **121**, 206–214.

Diepen, R., Engelhardt, F. & Smith-Agreda, V. (1954). Über Ort und Art der Entsehung des Neurosekretes im supra-optico-hypophysären System bei Hund und Katze. *Verh. anat. Ges. Munster* **1**, 276–286.

Eaton, A. G., Ferguson, F. P. & Beyer, F. T. (1946). The renal reabsorption of amino-acids in dogs: valine, leucine and isoleucine. *Am. J. Physiol.* **145**, 491–499.

Edwards, J. G. (1956). Efferent arterioles of glomeruli in the juxtamedullary zone of the human kidney. *Anat. Rec.* **125**, 521–529.

Edwards, J. G. & Condorelli, L. (1928). Studies on aglomerular and glomerular kidneys. *Am. J. Physiol.* **86**, 383–398.

Eigler, F. W. (1961). Short circuit measurements in proximal tubule of *Necturus* kidney. *Am. J. Physiol.* **201**, 157–163.

Eisner, G. M., Porusch, J. G., Goldstein, M. H. & Levitt, M. F. (1962). An appraisal of free water reabsorption in man. *J. Mt Sinai Hosp.* **29**, 38–49.

Faarup, P. (1965). On the morphology of the juxtaglomerular apparatus. *Acta anat.* **60**, 20–32.

Farquhar, M. G. & Palade, G. E. (1963). Junctional complexes in various epithelia. *J. cell Biol.* **17**, 375–412.

Ferguson, F. P., Eaton, A. G. & Ashman, J. S. (1947). Renal reabsorption of methionine in normal dog. *Proc. Soc. exp. Biol. Med. N.Y.* **66**, 582–585.

Feyel, P. & Vieillefosse, R. (1939). Les secrétions rénales de l'urée et des chlorures; études cytophysiologiques. *Archs. Anat. microsc.* **35**, 5–53.

Filehne, W. & Biberfeld, H. (1902). Beitrage zur Diurese. Einleitende Versuche, *Pflügers Arch. ges. Physiol.* **91**, 569–593.

Fisher, R. B. (1955). The absorption of water and of some small molecules from the isolated small intestine of the rat. *J. Physiol.* **130**, 655–664.

Fong, C. T. O., Schwartz, I. L., Popenoe, E. A., Silver, L. & Schoessler, M. A. (1959). On the molecular bonding of lysine-vasopressin at its renal receptor site. *Am. chem. J.* **81**, 2592–2593.

Fong, C. T. O., Silver, L., Christman, D. R. & Schwartz, I. L. (1960). On the mechanism of action of the antidiuretic hormone (vasopressin). *Proc. natn. Acad. Sci. U.S.A.* **46**, 1273–1277.

Fourman, J. (1966). Cholinesterase in the mammalian kidney. *Nature, Lond.* **209**, 812–813.

Frank, J. & Mayer, J. E. (1947). An osmotic diffusion pump. *Arch. Biochem.* **14**, 297–313.

Freeman, B., Livingston, A. E. & Richards, A. N. (1930). A second series of quantitative estimations of the concentration of chlorides in glomerular urine from frogs. *J. biol. Chem.* **87**, 467–477.

Fromageot, P. & Maier-Hüser, H. (1951). Obtention de vasopressin hautement active. *C. r. hebd. Séanc. Acad. Sci., Paris* **232**, 2367–2368.

Galan, E. (1949). Nephrosis in children. *Am. J. Dis. Child.* **77**, 328–337.

Ganote, C. E., Grantham, J. J., Moses, H. L., Burg, M. B. & Orloff, J. (1968). Ultrastructural studies of vasopressin effect on isolated perfused renal collecting tubules of the rabbit. *J. cell Biol.* **36**, 355–367.

Gertz, K. H. (1962). Direct measurement of the transtubular flux of electrolytes and non-electrolytes in the intact rat kidney. *Proc. XXII int. Congr. Physiol., Leiden,* **1**, 370–371.

— (1963). Transtubuläre Natriumchloridflüsse und Permeabilität für Nichtelecktrolyte im proximalen und distalen Konvolut der Rattenniere. *Pflügers Arch. ges. Physiol.* **276**, 336–356.

Gertz, K. H., Mangos, J. A., Braun, G. & Pagel, H. D. (1965). On the glomerular tubular balance in the rat kidney. *Pflügers Arch. ges. Physiol.* **285**, 360–372.

Gertz, K. H., Schmidt-Nielsen, B. & Pagel, D. (1966). Exchanges of water, urea and salt between the mammalian renal papilla and the surrounding urine. *Fedn Proc.* **25,** 327.

Giebisch, G., Klose, R. M. & Windhager, E. E. (1964). Micropuncture study of hypertonic sodium chloride loading in the rat. *Am. J. Physiol.* **206,** 687–693.

Giebisch, G. & Windhager, E. E. (1964). Renal tubular transfer of sodium, chloride and potassium. *Am. J. Med.* **36,** 643–669.

Ginetzinsky, A. G. (1958). Role of hyaluronidase in the reabsorption of water in the renal tubules: the mechanism of action of the antidiuretic hormone. *Nature, Lond.* **182,** 1218–1219.

Ginetzinsky, A. G., Broytman, A. I. & Ivanova, L. N. (1954). Gialuronidaznoya aktivnost mochi cheloveka. *Bjul. eksp. biol. med.* **38,** 37–40.

Ginetzinsky, A. G. & Ivanova, L. N. (1958). Rol sistemi gialurondvaya kistola-gialuronidaza v precese reabsorpeii vody v pochechuych kanaltsach. *Dokl. Akad. Nauk SSSR* **119,** 1043–1058.

Ginetzinsky, A. G., Krestinskaya, T. V., Natochin, Y., Sax, M. & Titova, L. (1960). Evolution of the substrate acted upon by antidiuretic hormone. *Physiologia bohemoslov.* **9,** 166–171.

Ginsburg, M. (1954). The secretion of antidiuretic hormone in response to haemorrhage and the fate of vasopressin in adrenalectomized rats. *J. Endocr.* **11,** 165–176.

Ginsburg, M. & Heller, H. (1953). The clearance of injected vasopressin from the circulation and its fate in the body. *J. Endocr.* **9,** 283–291.

Ginsburg, M. & Jayasena, K. (1968). The distribution of proteins that bind neurohypophysial hormones. *J. Physiol.* **197,** 65–76.

Glimstedt, G. (1942). Quantitativ histochemische Untersuchungen über die Niere. *Z. mikrosk-anat. Forsch.* **52,** 335–358.

Goffart, M. & Nys, J. (1965). Pouvoir de concentration du rein du paresseux (*Choleopus hoffmanni* Peters). *Archs int. Physiol.* **73,** 166–168.

Goldberg, M. & McCurdy, D. K. (1963). Factors determining maximum tubular reabsorption of water during the renal concentrating operation. *Clin. Res.* **11,** 408–420.

Goldman, A. G., Yallow, A. A. & Grossman, J. (1963). The kinetics of K^{42} distribution after intravenous administration in human subjects with particular reference to the kidney. *Clin. Sci.* **24,** 287–296.

Goodwin, H. E. & Kaufman, J. J. (1956). The renal lymphatics. *Urol. Surv.* **6,** 305–329.

Gottschalk, C. W. (1964). Osmotic concentration and dilution of the urine. *Am. J. Med.* **36,** 670–685.

Gottschalk, C. W., Lassiter, W. E. & Mylle, M. (1960). Localisation of urine acidification in the mammalian kidney. *Am. J. Physiol.* **198,** 581–585.

Gottschalk, C. W., Lassiter, W. E., Mylle, M., Ullrich, K. J., Schmidt-Neilsen, B., O'Dell, R. & Pehling, G. (1963). Micropuncture study of composition of loop of Henle fluid in desert rodents. *Am. J. Physiol.* **204,** 532–535.

Gottschalk, C. W. & Mylle, M. (1958). Micropuncture study of osmo-larity of renal tubular fluid in the hydropenic rat during osmotic diuresis. *Fedn Proc.* **17**, 58.

— (1959). Micropuncture study of the mammalian urinary concentrating mechanism: evidence for the counter-current hypothesis. *Am. J. Physiol.* **196**, 927–936.

Grantham, J. J. & Burg, M. B. (1966). Effect of vasopressin and cyclic AMP on permeability of isolated collecting tubules. *Am. J. Physiol.* **211**, 255–259.

Green, J. D. & Van Bremen, V. L. (1955). Electron microscopy of the pituitary and observations on neurosecretion. *Am. J. Anat.* **97**, 117–203.

Greenbaum, A. L. & Dicker, S. E. (1963a). The effects of mammalian posterior lobe hormones on the swelling of liver and kidney mito-chondria, in the rat and the dog. *Biochim. biophys. Acta* **74**, 519–524.

— (1963b). The swelling of mitochondria from the liver and kidney of a primitive rodent (*Aplodontia rufa*). *Biochem. biophys. Res. Commun.* **12**, 402–404.

Grünewald, P. & Popper, H. (1940). The histogenesis and physiology of the renal glomerulus in early postnatal life: histological examinations. *J. Urol.* **43**, 452–458.

Grünwald, M. F. (1909). Beitrage zur Physiologie und Pharmakologie der Niere. *Arch. exp. Path. Pharmak.* **60**, 360–383.

Guinnebault, M. & Morel, F. (1957). Rôle de la surrénale dans les mécanismes de la concentration de l'urine. *C. r. hebd. Séanc. Acad. Sci., Paris.* **244**, 2741–2745.

György, P., Keller, W. & Brehme, T. (1928). Nierenstoffweschel und Nierenentwicklung. *Biochem. Z.* **200**, 356–366.

Handler, J. S., Butcher, R. W., Sutherland, E. W. & Orloff, J. (1965). The effect of vasopressin and theophylline on the concentration of adenosine $3',5'$-phosphate in the urinary bladder of the toad. *J. biol. Chem.* **240**, 4524–4526.

Handler, J. S. & Orloff, J. (1963). Activation of phosphorylase in toad bladder and mammalian kidney by antidiuretic hormone. *Am. J. Physiol.* **205**, 298–302.

Handler, J. S., Petersen, M. & Orloff, J. (1966). Effect of metabolic inhibitors on the response of toad bladder to vasopressin. *Am. J. Physiol.* **211**, 1175–1180.

Hargitay, B. & Kuhn, W. (1951). Das multiplikationsprinzipals Grund-lage der Harnkonzentrierung in der Niere. *Z. Elektrochem.* **55**, 539–558.

Hargitay, B., Kuhn, W. & Wirz, H. (1951). Ein modellversuch zum Problem der Harnkonzentrierung. *Helv. physiol. pharmac. Acta.* **9**, C26.

Harvey, N., Jones, J. J. & Lee, J. (1967). The renal clearance and plasma binding of vasopressin in the dog. *J. Endocr.* **38**, 163–171.

Haynes, R. C. & Berthet, L. (1957). Studies on the mechanism of action of the adrenocorticotropic hormone. *J. biol. Chem.* **225**, 115–124.

Hays, R. M. & Leaf, A. (1962). Studies on the movement of water through the isolated toad bladder and its modification by vasopressin. *J. gen. Physiol.* **45**, 905–919.

Hayslett, J. P., Kashgarian, M. & Epstein, F. H. (1967). Changes in proximal and distal tubular reabsorption produced by rapid expansion of extracellular fluid. *J. clin. Invest.* **46**, 1254–1263.

Heller, H. (1937). The state in the blood and the excretion by the kidney of the antidiuretic principle of posterior pituitary extracts. *J. Physiol.* **89**, 81–95.

— (1944). The renal function of newborn infants. *J. Physiol.* **102**, 429–440.

— (1947a). Antidiuretic hormone in pituitary glands of newborn rats. *J. Physiol.* **106**, 28–32.

— (1947b). The response of newborn rats to administration of water by the stomach. *J. Physiol.* **106**, 245–255.

— (1949). Effects of dehydration on adult and newborn rats. *J. Physiol.* **108**, 303–314.

— (1952). The action and fate of vasopressin in newborn and infant rats. *J. Endocr.* **8**, 214–518.

— (1953). The fate and excretion of neurohypophysial principles. *J. Endocr.* **9**, 7–9P.

— (1954). Aspect of adrenal and pituitary function in the newborn. In *Neo-natal Studies* **8**, 31–47.

— (1957). The state and concentration of the neurohypophysial hormones in the blood. *Ciba Foundation Colloquia* on *Endocrinology* **11**, 8–14.

— (1960). Endocrine regulation of the metabolism of water: phylogenetic and ontogenetic aspects in: *The development of homeostasis with special reference to factors of the environment.* Symposium of the Czechoslovak Academy of Sciences, Prague, vol. 1, pp. 77–93.

Heller, H. & Lederis, K. (1959). Maturation of the hypothalamic-neurohypophysial system. *J. Physiol.* **147**, 299–314.

Heller, H. & Urban, F. F. (1935). The fate of the antidiuretic principle of post-pituitary extracts. *J. Physiol.* **85**, 502–518.

Heller, H. & Zaidi, S. M. (1957). The metabolism of exogenous and endogenous antidiuretic hormone in the kidney and liver *in vivo*. *Brit. J. Pharmac.* **12**, 284–292.

Heller, H. & Zaïmis, E. J. (1949). The antidiuretic and oxytocic hormones in the posterior pituitary glands of newborn infants and adults. *J. Physiol.* **109**, 162–169.

Heller, J. & Lojda, Z. (1960). The physiology of the antidiuretic hormone—VIII. Histological note on Ginetzinsky's theory of the action of antidiuretic hormone. *Physiologia bohemoslov.* **6**, 504–509.

Henderson, V. E. (1905). The factors of the ureter pressure. *J. Physiol.* **33**, 175–188.

Henry, L. P., Keyl, M. J. & Bell R. D. (1969). Flow and protein concentration of capsular renal lymph in the conscious dog. *Am. J. Physiol.* **217**, 411–413.

Herd, J. A., Hollenberg, M., Thoburn, G. D., Kopald, H. H. & Barger, A. C. (1962). Myocardial blood flow determined with [85]Kr in unanaesthetised dogs. *Am. J. Physiol.* **203**, 122–129.

Herrera, F. C. (1966). Action of ouabain on sodium transport in the toad urinary bladder. *Am. J. Physiol.* **210**, 980–986.

Hilger, H. H., Klümper, J. D. & Ullrich, K. J. (1958). Wasser-rück-resorption und ionen transport durch die Sammel-röhrzellen der Saügetiere. *Pflügers Arch. ges. Physiol.* **267**, 218–237.

Hirokawa, W. (1908). Uber den osmotischen Druck des Nierenparen-chyms. *Beitr. chem. Physiol. Path.* **11**, 458–470.

Höber, B. (1947). *Physical Chemistry of Cells and Tissues.* London: Churchill.

Horster, M., Schnermann, J. & Thurau, K. (1969). The function of juxtamedullary nephrons in water diuresis and ADH induced antidiuresis. *Proc. 6th Meeting Soc. Nephrology, Vienna* (in the press).

Horster, M. & Thurau, K. (1968). Micropuncture studies on the filtration rate of single superficial and juxtamedullary glomeruli in the rat kidney. *Pflügers Arch. ges. Physiol.* **301**, 162–181.

House, F., Pfeiffer, F. & Braun, H. (1963). Influence of diet on urine concentration in *Aplodontia rufa* and the rabbit. *Nature, Lond.* **199**, 181–182.

Hüber, G. C. (1917). A method for isolating the renal tubules of mammalia. *Anat. Rec.* **5**, 187–194.

Hummel, R. (1963). Untersuchungen über den Elektrolyt- und Wasserhaushalt von *Meriones Shawii Shawii* (Duvernoy). *Helv. physiol. pharmac. Acta.* Suppl. **14**, 1–76.

Ishida, Y. & Hara, K. (1964). Studies on the inhibitory actions of synthetic peptides on the effects of oxytocin and vasopressin. *Chem. Pharm. Bull.* **12**, 872–880.

Jamison, R. L., Bennett, C. M. & Berliner, R. W. (1967). Countercurrent multiplication by the thin loop of Henle. *Am. J. Physiol.* **212**, 357–366.

Jarausch, K. H. & Ullrich, K. J. (1957). Zur Technik der Enthnahme von Harnproben aus einzelnen Sammelröhren der Saügetiereniere mittels Polyäthylincapillaren. *Pflügers Arch. ges. Physiol.* **264**, 88–94.

Jones, A. M. & Schlapp, W. (1936). The action and fate of injected posterior pituitary extracts in the decapitated cat. *J. Physiol.* **87**, 144–157.

Jones, W. H. S. (1923). *Ancient medicine.* Vol. 1. London: Heinemann.

Kaplan, A., Freidman, H. E. & Kruger, H. E. (1942). Observations concerning the origin of renal lymph. *Am. J. Physiol.* **138**, 553–556.

Kashgarian, M., Stoeckle, H., Gottschalk, C. W. & Ullrich, K. J. (1963). Transtubular electrochemical potentials of sodium and chloride in proximal and distal tubules of rats during antidiuresis and water diuresis (diabetes insipidus). *Pflügers Arch. ges. Physiol.* **277**, 86–106.

Kaye, G. I., Wheeler, H. O., Whitlock, R. T. & Lane, N. (1966). Fluid transport in the rabbit gall-bladder. *J. cell Biol.* **30**, 237–243.

Kedem, O. & Katchalsky, A. (1958). Thermodynamic analysis of the permeability of biological membranes to non-electrolytes. *Biochim. biophys. Acta* **27**, 229–246.

Kelman, R. B. (1962). A theoretical note on exponential flow in the proximal part of the mammalian nephron. *Bull. math. Biophys.* **24**, 303–317.

— (1965). Mathematical analysis of sodium reabsorption in proximal part of nephron in presence of nonreabsorbed solute. *J. theor. Biol.* **8**, 22–26.

Kittelson, J. A. (1917). The postnatal growth of the kidney of the albino rat, with observations on an adult human kidney. *Anat. Rec.* **13**, 385–408.

Klein, E., Burdon-Sanderson, J., Foster, M. & Brunton, T. L. (1873). *Handbook for the Physiological Laboratory.* London: Churchill.

Klümper, J. D., Ullrich, K. J. & Hilger, H. H. (1958). Das Verhalten des Harnstoffs in den Sammelröhren der Saügetierniere. *Pflügers Arch. ges. Physiol.* **267**, 238–243.

Koefoed-Johnsen, V. & Ussing, H. H. (1953). The contributions of diffusion and flow to the passage of D_2O through living membranes. *Acta physiol. Scand.* **28**, 60–76.

Koike, T. I. & Kellogg, R. H. (1963). Effect of urea loading on urine osmolality during osmotic diuresis in hydropenic rats. *Am. J. Physiol.* **205**, 1053–1057.

Kramer, K. (1962). Medullary blood flow and the countercurrent system. *Proc. XXII int. Congr. Physiol., Leiden*, **1**, 381–383.

Kramer, K. & Deetjen, P. (1961). Sodium reabsorption and oxygen consumption in the mammalian kidney. *Proc. 1st int. Congr. Nephrology, Geneva*, Evian. 687.

Kramer, K., Deetjen, P. & Brechtelsbauer, H. (1961). Gegenstromdiffusion des Sauerstoffs im Nierenmark. *Pflügers Arch. ges. Physiol.* **274**, 63C.

Kramer, K., Thurau, K. & Deetjen, P. (1960). Hämodynamik des Nierensmarks. Capilläre Passagezeit, Blutvolumen, Durchblutung, Gewebshämatocrit und O_2 Verbrauch dies Nierenmarks *in situ*. *Pflügers Arch. ges. Physiol.* **270**, 251–269.

Kuhn, W. & Martin, H. (1941). Temperaturabhängigkeit der Adsorbierbarkeit als mittel zur laufenden Fraktionierung oder Konzentrierung von Lösungen. *Z. phys. Chem.* (A) **189**, 317–326.

Kuhn, W. & Ramel, L. (1959). Aktiver Salztransport als möglicher (und warscheinlicher) Einzeleffekt bei der Harnkonzentrierung in der Niere. *Helv. chim. Acta* **42**, 628–660.

Kuhn, W. & Ryffel, K. (1942). Herstellung konzentriereter Lösungen aus verdünnten durch blosse Membranwirkung. Ein Modelverzuch zur funktion der Niere. *Hoppe Seyler's Z. physiol. Chem.* **276**, 145–178.

Lamdin, E. (1959). Mechanisms of urinary concentration and dilution. *A.M.A. Archs int. Med.* **103**, 644–671.

Lampen, J. O., Arnow, P. M., Borowska, Z. & Laskin, A. I. (1962). Location and role of sterol at nystatin-binding sites. *J. Bact.* **84,** 1152–1155.

Lampen, J. O., Arnow, P. M. & Safferman, R. S. (1960). Mechanism of protection by sterols against polyene antibiotics. *J. Bact.* **80,** 200–208.

Landwehr, D. M., Klose, R. M. & Giebisch, G. (1947). Renal tubular sodium and water reabsorption in the isotonic sodium chloride loaded rat. *Am. J. Physiol.* **212,** 1327–1333.

Lapp, H. & Nolte, A. (1962). Vergleichende elektronen mikroskopische Untersuchungen am Mark der Rattenniere bei Harnkonzentrierung und Harnverdunnung. *Frankfurt Z. Path.* **7,** 617–633.

Larson, E. (1938). Tolerance and fate of the pressor principle of posterior pituitary extracts in anaesthetised animals. *J. Pharmac.* **62,** 346–352.

Lassen, N. A. & Longley, J. B. (1961). Countercurrent exchange in vessels of renal medulla. *Proc. Soc. exp. Biol. Med.* **106,** 743–748.

Lassiter, W. E., Gottschalk, C. W. & Mylle, M. (1960). Composition of loop of Henle and collecting duct fluids in the hamster papilla. *Fedn Proc.* **19,** 369.

— (1961). Micropuncture study of net transtubular movement of water and urea in non-diuretic mammalian kidney. *Am. J Physiol.* **200,** 1139–1146.

Lassiter, W. E., Mylle, M. & Gottschalk, C. W. (1964). Net transtubular movement of water and urea in saline diuresis. *Am. J. Physiol.* **206,** 664–673.

Lauson, H. D. (1967). Metabolism of antidiuretic hormones. *Am. J. Med.* **42,** 713–744.

Lauson, H. D., Bocanegra, M. & Beuzeville, C. F. (1965). Hepatic and renal clearance of vasopressin from plasma of dogs. *Am. J. Physiol.* **209,** 199–214.

Leaf, A. (1960). Some actions of neurohypophysial hormone on a living membrane. *J. gen. Physiol.* **43,** 175–189.

— (1965). Transepithelial transport and its hormonal control in the toad bladder. *Ergebn. Physiol.* **56,** 216–228.

Leaf, A. & Dempsey, E. (1960). Some effects of mammalian neurohypophysial hormones on metabolism and active transport of sodium by the isolated toad bladder. *J. biol. Chem.* **235,** 2160–2164.

Leaf, A. & Hays, R. M. (1962). Permeability of the toad bladder to solutes and its modification by vasopressin. *J. gen. Physiol.* **45,** 921–932.

Leaf, A., Kerr, W. S., Wrong, O. & Chatillon, J. Y. (1954). Effect of graded compression of the renal artery on water and solute excretion. *Am. J. Physiol.* **179,** 191–200.

Lechêne, C., Corby, C. & Morel, F. (1966). Distribution des néphrons accessibles à la surface du rein en fonction de la longueur de leur anse de Henle chez le Rat, le Hamster, le Mérion et le Psammonys. *C. r. hebd. Séanc. Acad. Sci., Paris.* **262,** 1126–1130.

Lehninger, A. L. & Neubert, D. (1961). Effect of oxytocin, vasopressin and other disulfide hormones on uptake and extrusion of water by mitochondria. *Proc. natn. Acad. Sci.* U.S.A. **47**, 1929–1936.

Lever, A. F. (1965). The vasa recta and countercurrent multiplication *Acta. med. scand. Suppl.* **434**, 1–43.

Leyssac, P. P. (1963). The *in vivo* effect of angiotensin on the proximal tubular reabsorption of salt in rat kidneys. *Acta. physiol. scand.* **58**, 236–242.

Lichtenstein, N. A. & Leaf, A. (1965). Effect of amphotericin B on the permeability of toad bladder. *J. clin. Invest.* **10**, 1328–1342.

— (1966). Evidence for a double series permeability barrier at the mucosal surface of the toad bladder. *Ann. N.Y. Acad. Sci.* **137**, 556–565.

Lichtfield, J. B. & Bott, P. A. (1962). Micropuncture study of renal excretion of water, K, Na and Cl in the rat. *Am. J. Physiol.* **203**, 667–670.

Ljungberg, F. (1947). On the reabsorption of chlorides in the kidney of the rabbit. *Acta. med. scand. Suppl.* **186**, 1–189.

Ljungquist, A. (1964). Structure of the arteriole–glomerular units in different zones of the kidney. *Nephron* **1**, 329–333.

Longley, J. B., Banfield, W. G. & Brindley, D. C. (1959). Structure of the rete mirabile in the kidney of the rat as seen with the electron-microscope. *J. biophys. biochem. Cytol.* **7**, 103–105.

Longley, J. B. & Fisher, E. R. (1956). A histochemical basis for changes in renal tubular function in young mice. *Qt. Jl. Microsc. Sci.* **97**, 187–195.

Longley, J. B., Lassen, N. A. & Lilienfield, L. S. (1958). Tracer studies on renal medullary circulation. *Fedn Proc.* **17**, 99.

MacRobbie, E. A. C. & Ussing, H. H. (1961). Osmotic behaviour of the epithelial cells of frog skin. *Acta physiol. scand.* **53**, 348–359.

Maffly, R. H., Hays, R. M., Lamdin, E. & Leaf, A. (1960). The effect of neurohypophysial hormones on the permeability of the toad bladder to urea. *J. clin. Invest.* **39**, 630–641.

Maier-Hüser, H., Clauser, H., Fromageot, P. & Plongeron, R. (1953). Préparations des hormones du lobe postérieur de l'hypophyse de boeuf. *Biochim. biophys. Acta* **11**, 252–257.

Malnic, G., Klose, R. M. & Giebisch, G. (1966a). Micropuncture study of distal tubular potassium and sodium transport in rat nephron. *Am. J. Physiol.* **211**, 529–547.

— (1966b). Micropuncture study of distal tubular potassium and sodium transfer in rat kidney. *Am. J. Physiol.* **211**, 548–559.

Malvin, R. L. & Wilde, W. S. (1959). Washout of renal countercurrent Na gradient by osmotic diuresis. *Am. J. Physiol.* **197**, 177–180.

Malvin, R. L., Wilde, W. S. & Sullivan, L. P. (1958). Localisation of nephron transport by stop flow analysis. *Am. J. Physiol.* **194**, 132–142.

March, D. J. & Solomon, S. (1965). Analysis of electrolyte movement in thin Henle's loops of hamster papilla. *Am. J. Physiol.* **208**, 1119–1128.

Marshall, E. K. (1930). A comparison of the function of the glomerular and aglomerular kidney. *Am. J. Physiol.* **94**, 1–14.

Marshall, E. K. & Smith, H. W. (1930). The glomerular development of the vertebrate kidney in relation to habitat. *Biol. Bull. mar. biol. Lab. Woods Hole.* **59**, 135–144.

Martin, H. & Kuhn, W. (1941a). Multiplikationsverfahren zur Spaltung von Racematen. *Z. Elektrochem.* **47**, 216–220.

— (1941b). Multiplikationsverfahren zur Trennung von Gasgemischen, insbesondere bei Anwendung von Schwerefeldern. *Z. phys. Chem.* **189**, 219–316.

Maude, D. L., Shehadeh, I. & Solomon, A. K. (1966). Sodium and water transport in single perfused distal tubules of *Necturus* kidney. *Am. J. Physiol.* **211**, 1043–1049.

Maximow, A. A. & Bloom, W. (1952). *A Textbook of Histology*, vol. 1. Philadelphia: Saunders.

Mayer, F. S. (1960). Identification of the antidiuretic substance in human urine. *Acta endocr.* **35**, 568–574.

McCance, R. A. (1948). Renal function in early life. *Physiol. Rev.* **28**, 331–348.

McCance, R. A., Naylor, N. J. B. & Widdowson, E. M. (1954). The response of infants to a large dose of water. *Arch. Dis. Childh.* **29**, 104–109.

McCance, R. A. & Stanier, M. W. (1960). The function of the metanephros of foetal rabbits and pigs. *J. Physiol.* **151**, 479–483.

McCance, R. A. & Widdowson, E. M. (1953). Normal and abnormal aspects of renal function in early life. *Ber. phys. med. Ges. Wurzburg* **66**, 115–135.

— (1954). The effect of birth on renal function. *Modern Problems in Pediatrics*, vol. 1, 145–150. Basle: Karger.

McCance, R. A. & Wilkinson, E. (1947). The response of adult and suckling rats to the administration of water and hypertonic solutions of urea and salt. *J. Physiol.* **106**, 256–263.

McKenna, O. C. & Angelakos, E. T. (1968). Adrenergic innervation of the canine kidney. *Circulation Res.* **22**, 345–354.

Metz, B. (1959). Données récentes sur la régulation thermique. *J. Physiol. Paris.* **51**, 263–318.

Moffat, D. B. (1967). The fine structure of the blood vessels of the renal medulla with particular reference to the control of the medullary circulation. *Ultrastruct. Res.* **19**, 523–537.

Moffat, D. B. & Fourman, J. (1963). The vascular pattern of the rat kidney. *J. Anat.* **97**, 543–553.

Montgomery, H. (1935). Quantitative studies of the composition of glomerular urine—XII. The reaction of glomerular urine of frogs and Necturi. *J. biol. Chem.* **110**, 749–761.

Morel, F. (1955). Les modalités de l'excrétion du potassium par le rein: étude expérimentale à l'aide du radio-potassium chez le lapin. *Helv. physiol. pharmac. Acta* **13**, 276–294.

Morel, F. & Guinnebault, M. (1961). Les mécanismes de concentration et de dilution de l'urine. *J. Physiol., Paris* **53**, 75–130.

Morel, F., Guinnebault, M. & Amiel, C. (1960). Mise en évidence d'un processus d'échange d'eau par contre courant dans les régions profondes du rein du Hamster. *Helv. physiol. pharmac. Acta* **18,** 183–192.

Morel, F. & Jard, S. (1963). Inhibition of frog (*Rana esculenta*) antidiuretic action of vasotocin by some analogues. *Am. J. Physiol.* **204,** 227–232.

Morgan, T. & Berliner, R. W. (1969). A study by continuous microperfusion of water and electrolyte movements in the loop of Henle and distal tubule in the rat. *Nephron* **6,** 388–405.

Morgan, T., Sakai, F. & Berliner, R. W. (1968). *In vitro* permeability of medullary collecting ducts to water and urea. *Am. J. Physiol.* **214,** 574–581.

Mudge, G. H., Foulks, J. & Gilman, A. (1949). Effect of urea diuresis on renal excretion of electrolytes. *Am. J. Physiol.* **158,** 218–230.

Munkacsi, I. & Palkovits, M. (1965). Volumetric analysis of glomerular size in kidneys of mammals living in desert, semi-desert or water-rich environment in the Sudan. *Circulation Res.* **17,** 303–311

Nanninga, L. B., Swann, H. G. & Schubert, M. L. (1962). Outflow patterns of indicator dye continuously injected into tubes with laminar outflow. *Tex. Rep. Biol. Med.* **20,** 384–396.

Natochin, J. V. & Shakhmatova, E. I. (1968). The role of intercellular substance and hyaluronidase in the increase of permeability of frog urinary bladder induced by antidiuretic hormone. *Endocr. Exp.* **2,** 151–160.

Nilson, O. (1965). The adrenergic innervation of the kidney. *Lab. Invest.* **14,** 1392–1395.

Nungesser, W. C. & Pfeiffer, E. W. (1965). Water balance and maximum concentrating capacity in the primitive rodent, *Aplodontia rufa. Comp. Biochem. Physiol.* **14,** 289–297.

Nungesser, W. C., Pfeiffer, E. W., Iverson, D. A. & Wallerius, J. F. (1960). Evaluation of renal countercurrent hypothesis in *Aplodontia. Fedn Proc.* **19,** 362.

Ochwadt, B. K. & Pitts, R. F. (1956). Disparity between phenol red and diodrast clearances in the dog. *Am. J. Physiol.* **187,** 318–322.

O'Connor, W. J. (1950). The role of the neurohypophysis of the dog in determining urinary changes, and the antidiuretic activity of urine, following the administration of sodium chloride or urea. *Q. Jl. exp. Physiol.* **36,** 21–47.

— (1962), *Renal Function*. Monographs of the Physiological Society, No. 10. London: Edward Arnold.

O'Dell, R. & Schmidt-Nielsen, B. (1960). Concentrating ability and kidney structure. *Fedn Proc.* **19,** 366.

Opie, E. L. (1949). Movement of water in tissues removed from the body and its relation to movements of water during life. *J. exp. Med.* **89,** 185–208.

Orloff, J. & Burg, M. B. (1960). Vasopressin resistant diabetes insipidus, In *The Metabolic Basis of Inherited Disease*. New York: McGraw-Hill.

Orloff, J. & Handler, J. S. (1964). The cellular mode of action of antidiuretic hormone. *Am. J. Med.* **36**, 686–694.

— (1967). The role of adenosine 3',5'-phosphate in the action of antidiuretic hormone. *Am. J. Med.* **42**, 757–768.

Orr, J. & Snaith, A. H. (1959). A method for the estimation of antidiuretic hormone in urine. *J. Endocr.* **18**, 16P.

Oswaldo, L. & Latta, H. (1966). The thin limbs of the loop of Henle. *J. ultrastr. Res.* **15**, 144–168.

Owen, E. E. & Robinson, R. R. (1964). Urea production and excretion by the chicken kidney. *Am. J. Physiol.* **206**, 1321–1326.

Page, L. B. & Reem, G. H. (1952). Urinary concentration mechanism in the dog. *Am. J. Physiol.* **171**, 572–581.

Page, L. B., Scott-Baker, J. C., Zak, G. A., Becker, E. L. & Baxter, C. F. (1954). Effect of variation in filtration rate on the urinary concentrating mechanism in the seal, *Phoca vitulina. J. cell. comp. Physiol.* **43**, 257–269.

Pak Poy, R. K. & Bentley, P. J. (1960). Fine structure of the epithelial cells of the toad urinary bladder. *Expl Cell Res.* **20**, 235–237.

Papez, J. W. (1940). The fine structure of the neurohypophysis. In *Ultrastructure and Cellular Chemistry of Neural Tissue*, Ed. WALSCH, H. London: Cassell.

Pappenheimer, J. R. (1953). Passage of molecules through capillary vessels. *Physiol. Rev.* **23**, 387–423.

Pappenheimer, J. R., Renkin, E. M. & Borrero, L. M. (1951). Filtration, diffusion and molecular sieving through peripheral capillary membranes. *Am. J. Physiol.* **167**, 13–46.

Parsons, D. S. & Wingate, D. L. (1961). The effect of osmotic gradients on fluid transfer across rat intestine *in vitro. Biochim. biophys. Acta* **46**, 170–176.

Payne, J. F. (1897). Harvey and Galen. *The Harveyan Oration*. London: Frowde.

Peachey, L. D. & Rasmussen, H. (1961). Structure of the toad's urinary bladder as related to its physiology. *J. biophys. biochem. Cytol.* **10**, 529–532.

Peter, K. (1909). DIE NIERENKANALCHEN DES MENSCHEN UND EINIGER SAÜGETIERE. In *Untersuchungen über Bau und Entwickelung der Niere*, ed. PETER, K. vol. 1, pp. 335–336. Jena: Gustav Fischer.

— (1927). *Untersuchungen über Bau und Entwicklung der Niere*. Jena: Gustav Fischer.

Petersen, M. J. & Edelman, I. S. (1964). Calcium inhibition of the action of vasopressin on the urinary bladder of the toad. *J. clin. Invest.* **45**, 583–592.

Pfeiffer, E. W. (1968). Comparative anatomical observations of the mammalian renal pelvis and medulla. *J. Anat.* **102**, 321–331.

Pfeiffer, E. W., Nungesser, W. C., Iverson, D. A. & Wallerius, J. F. (1960). The renal anatomy of the primitive rodent, *Aplodontia rufa*, and a consideration of its functional significance. *Anat. Rec.* **137**, 227–235.

Pierce, J. A. & Montgomery, H. (1935). A microquinhydrone electrode: its application to the determination of the pH of glomerular urine of *Necturus. J. biol. Chem.* **110**, 763–775.

Pilkington, L. A., Binder, R., de Haas, J. C. M. & Pitts, R. F. (1965). Intrarenal distribution of blood flow. *Am. J. Physiol.* **208**, 1107–1113.

Pinter, G. G. & Shohet, J. L. (1963). Origin of sodium concentration profile in the renal medulla. *Nature, Lond.* **200**, 954–958.

Pitts, R. F. (1959). *The Physiological Basis of Diuretic Therapy.* Springfield: Charles C Thomas.

— (1963). *Physiology of the Kidney and Body Fluids.* Chicago: Year Book Medical Publishers.

Pitts, R. F., Brown, J. L. & Samiy, A. H. E. (1959). The site of renal tubular reabsorption of amino-acids. *Proc. XXIst int. Physiol Congr. B.A.* 213.

Plakke, R. K. & Pfeiffer, E. W. (1964). Blood vessels of the mammalian renal medulla. *Science* **146**, 1683–1685.

— (1965). Influence of plasma urea on urine concentration in the opossum (*Didelphis marsupialis virginiana*). *Nature, Lond.* **207**, 866–867.

Pliška, V., Rudinger, J., Douša, T. & Cort, J. H. (1968). Oxytocin activity and the integrity of the disulphide bridge. *Am. J. Physiol.* **215**, 916–920.

Pomeranz, B. H., Birtch, A. G. & Barger, A. C. (1968). Neural control of intrarenal blood flow. *Am. J. Physiol.* **215**, 1067–1081.

Potter, E. L. (1946). Bilateral renal agenesis. *J. Pediat.* **29**, 68–75.

Puschett, J. B. & Goldberg, M. (1968). The acute effects of furosemide on acid and electrolyte excretion in man. *J. Lab. clin. Med.* **71**, 666–677.

Ramsay, J. A. (1949). A new method of freezing point determination for small quantities. *J. exp. Biol.* **26**, 57–64.

Ramsay, J. A. & Brown, R. H. J. (1955). Simplified apparatus and procedure for freezing point determinations upon small volumes of fluid. *J. scient. instrum.* **32**, 372–375.

Rasmussen, H. & Schwartz, L. I. (1964). Studies of the interaction between neurohypophysial hormones and the amphibian urinary bladder. In *Oxytocin, Vasopressin and their Structural Analogues.* London: Pergamon Press.

Rasmussen, H., Schwartz, I. L., Schoessler, M. A. & Hochster, G. (1960). Studies on the mechanism of action of vasopressin. *Proc. natn Acad. Sci. U.S.A.* **46**, 1278–1287.

Rasmussen, H., Schwartz, I. L., Young, R. & Marc-Aurele, J. (1963). Structural requirements for the action of neurohypophysial hormones upon the isolated amphibian urinary bladder. *J. gen. physiol.* **46**, 1171–1189.

Rector, F. C., Brunner, F. P. & Seldin, D. W. (1966). Mechanism of glomerulotubular balance—I. Effect of aortic constriction and elevated uretero-pelvic pressure on glomerular filtration rate, fractional reabsorption, transit time, and tubular size in the proximal tubule of the rat. *J. clin. Invest.* **45**, 590–602.

Rennie, D. W., Reeves, R. B. & Pappenheimer, J. R. (1958). Oxygen pressure and its relation to intrarenal blood flow. *Am. J. Physiol.* **195**, 120–132.

Ressler, C. & Rachelle, J. R. (1958). Further properties of isoglutamine-oxytocin; inhibition of pressor activity of vasopressin. *Proc. Soc. exp. Biol. Med.* **98**, 170–172.

Reubi, F. (1958). Objections à la théorie de la séparation intrarénale des hématies et du plasma (Pappenheimer). *Helv. med. Acta* **25**, 516–523.

Rhodin, J. A. G. (1958). Anatomy of kidney tubules. *Int. Rev. Cytol.* **7**, 485–534.

Rhodin, J. A. G. (1965). Fine structure of the peritubular capillaries of the human kidney, in *Progress in Pyelonephritis*. Philadelphia: Davis.

Richards, A. N. (1929). *Methods and Results of Investigations of the Function of the Kidney*. Baltimore: Williams & Wilkins.

— (1934). Processes of urine formation in the amphibian kidney. *Harvey Lec.* **30**, 93–118.

Richards, A. N. & Walker, A. M. (1936). Methods of collecting fluid from known regions of the renal tubules of amphibia and of perfusing the lumen of a single tubule. *Am. J. Physiol.* **118**, 111–120.

Robbins, E. & Mauro, A. (1960). Experimental study of the independence of diffusion and hydrodynamic permeability coefficients in collodion membranes. *J. gen. Physiol.* **43**, 523–532.

Robinson, J. R. (1950). Osmoregulation in surviving cells from the kidneys of adult rats. *Proc. Roy. Soc. B* **137**, 378–402.

— (1960). Metabolism of intracellular water. *Physiol. Rev.* **40**, 112–149.

Rodeck, H. (1958). Neurosekretion und Wasserhaushalt bei Neugeborenen und Säuglingen. *Arch. Kinderheilk.* **36**, 1–62.

Rodeck, H. & Caesar, R. (1956). Zur Entwicklung der Neurosekretorischen Systems bei Saügern und Mensch und der Regulations-mechanism des Wasserhaushaltes. *Z. Zellforsch. mikrosk. Anat.* **44**, 666–691.

Rudinger, J. & Jošt, K. (1964a). Synthetic analogues of oxytocin: structural relations. In *Oxytocin, Vasopressin and their Structural Analogues*. London: Pergamon Press.

— (1964b). A biologically active analogue of oxytocin not containing a disulfide group. *Experientia* **20**, 570–571.

Ruiz-Guinazu, A., Arrizurieta, E. E. & Yelinek, L. (1964). Electrolyte, water and urea content in dog kidneys in different states of diuresis. *Am. J. Physiol.* **206**, 725–730.

Ruiz-Guinazu, A., Pehling, G., Rumrich, G. & Ullrich, K. J. (1961). Glucose- und Milchsäurekonzentration an der Spitze des vascularen Gegenstromsystems in Nieremark. *Pflügers Arch. ges. Physiol.* **274**, 311–317.

Rytand, D. R. (1938). The number and size of mammalian glomeruli as related to kidney and body weight, with methods for their ennumeration and measurements. *Am. J. Anat.* **62**, 507–520.

Sakai, F., Jamison, R. L. & Berliner, R. W. (1965). A method for exposing the rat renal medulla *in vivo*: micropuncture of the collecting duct. *Am. J. Physiol.* **209**, 663–668.

Santos-Martinez, J. & Selkurt, E. E. (1969). Renal lymph and its relationship to the countercurrent multiplier system of the kidney. *Am. J. Physiol.* **216**, 1548–1555.

Sawyer, W. H. (1963). Neurohypophysial peptides and water excretion in the vertebrate. *Mem. Soc. Endocr.* **13**, 45–58.

Sawyer, W. H. & Valtin, H. (1965). Inhibition of vasopressin antidiuresis by extracts of pituitaries from rats with hereditary hypothalamic diabetes insipidus and by oxytocin. *Endocrinology* **76**, 999–1001.

Scaglione, P. R., Dell, R. B. & Winters, R. W. (1965). Lactate concentration in the medulla of rat kidney. *Am. J. Physiol.* **209**, 1193–1198.

Scharrer, E. (1954). The maturation of the hypothalamic–hypophysial neurosecretory system in the dog. *Anat. Rec.* **118**, 437.

Schmidt-Nielsen, B. (1962). Movements of urea in the renal countercurrent system. *XXII Int. Congr. Physiol. Leiden*, vol. 1, pp. 377–380. Intern. Congress Series, Amsterdam.

Schmidt-Nielsen, B. & O'Dell, R. (1959). Distribution and active uptake of urea in renal tissue. *Fedn. Proc.* **18**, 138.

— (1960). Functional distribution of solutes in the renal tissue of rodents. *Fedn. Proc.* **19**, 366.

Schmidt-Nielsen, B., Schmidt-Nielsen, K., Brokaw, A. & Schneiderman, H. (1948). Water conservation in desert rodents. *J. cell. comp. Physiol.* **32**, 331–360.

Schmidt-Nielsen, B. & Shrauger, C. R. (1963). Handling of urea and related compounds by the renal tubules of the frog. *Am. J. Physiol.* **205**, 483–488

Schmidt-Nielsen, B., Ullrich, K. J., O'Dell, R., Pehling G., Gottschalk, C. W., Lassiter, W. E. & Mylle, M. (1960). Micropuncture study of the composition of fluid from cortical nephrons in the rat kidney. *Excerpta med.* 29–72.

Schmidt-Nielsen, K. (1964). *Desert Animals. Physiological Problems of Heat and Water.* Oxford: Clarendon Press.

Schnermann, J. (1968). Microperfusion study of single short loops of Henle in rat kidney. *Pflüger's Arch. ges. Physiol.* **300**, 255–282.

Schnermann, J., Nagel, W. & Thurau, K. (1966). Die frühdistale Natrium-konzentration in Rattennieren nach renale Ischämic und haemorrhagischer Hypotension. *Pflügers Arch. ges. Physiol.* **287**, 296–304.

Schoen, A. (1969). Water conservation and the structure of the kidneys of tropical bovids. *J. Physiol.* **204**, 143P.

Scholander, P. F. (1954). Secretion of gases against high pressures in the swimbladder of deep sea fishes. The *rete mirabile. Biol. Bull. mar. biol. lab. Woods Hole* **107**, 260–277.

— (1957). The wonderful net. *Scient. Am.* **196**, 96–107.

— (1958). Countercurrent exchange: a principle in biology. *Hvalvadets Skrifter.* **44**, 1–24.

Scholander, P. F. & Schevill, W. E. (1955). Countercurrent vascular heat exchanges in the fins of whales. *J. appl. Physiol.* **8**, 279-282.

Schwartz, I. L., Rasmussen, H., Livingston, L. M. & Marc-Aurele, J. (1964). Neurohypophysial hormone-receptor interaction. In *Oxytocin, Vasopressin and their Structural Analogues*. London: Pergamon Press.

Schwartz, I. L., Rasmussen, H. & Rudinger, J. (1964). Activity of neurohypophysial hormone analogues lacking a disulfide bridge. *Proc. Natn. Acad. Sci. U.S.A.* **52**, 1044–1045.

Schwartz, I. L., Rasmussen, H., Schoessler, M. A., Silver, L. & Fong, C. T. O. (1960). Relation of chemical attachment to physiological action of vasopressin. *Proc. Natn. Acad. Sci. U.S.A.* **46**, 1288–1295.

Schwartz, I. L., & Walter, R. (1965). Factors influencing the reactivity of the toad bladder to the hydro-osmotic action of vasopressin. *Am. J. Med.* **42**, 769–776.

Selkurt, E. E. (1954). Sodium excretion by the mammalian kidney. *Physiol. Rev.* **34**, 287–333.

— (1963). The renal circulation. In *Handbook of Physiology. Circulation*. Washington: *Am. Physiol. Soc.*

Sellwood, R. V. & Verney, E. B. (1955). The effect of water and of isotonic saline administration on the renal plasma and glomerular filtrate flows in the dog, with incidental observations of the effects on these flows of compression of the carotid and renal arteries. *Phil. Trans. R. Soc.* **B238**, 361–396.

Shannon, J. A. (1938). The renal reabsorption and excretion of urea under conditions of extreme diuresis. *Am. J. Physiol.* **122**, 782–791.

— (1942). The control of renal excretion of water. The effect of variations in the state of hydration on water excretion in dogs with diabetes insipidus. *J. exp. Med.* **76**, 371–386.

Siebeck, R. (1912). Uber die osmotischen Eigenschaften der Niere. *Pflüger's Arch. ges. Physiol.* **148**, 443–521.

Skadhauge, E. (1969). The mechanism of salt and water absorption in the intestine of the eel (*Anguilla Anguilla*) adapted to waters of various salinities. *J. Physiol.* **204**, 135–158.

Skadhauge, E. & Schmidt-Nielsen, B. (1967). Renal medullary electrolyte and urea gradient in chickens and turkeys. *Am. J. Physiol.* **212**, 1313–1318.

Smith, C. A. (1951). *The Physiology of the Newborn Infant*. Springfield, Illinois: C. Thomas.

Smith, H. W. (1930). The absorption and excretion of water and salts by marine teleosts. *Am. J. Physiol.* **93**, 480–487.

— (1937). *The Physiology of the Kidney*. London: Oxford University Press.

— (1943). *Lectures on the Kidney*. University Extension Division: University of Kansas, Lawrence, Kansas.

— (1947). The excretion of water. *Bull. N.Y. Acad. Med.* **23**, 177–195.

— (1951). *The Kidney: Structure and Function in Health and Disease*. New York: Oxford University Press.

— (1952). Renal excretion of sodium and water. *Fedn Proc.* **11**, 701–705.

— (1956). *Principles of Renal Physiology*. New York: Oxford University Press.

Smith, H. W. (1959). The fate of sodium and water in the renal tubules. *Bull. N.Y. Acad. Med.* **35,** 293–316.

Smith, M. W. & Sachs, H. (1961). Inactivation of arginine – vasopressin by rat kidney slices. *Biochem. J.* **79,** 663–669.

Smith, M. W. & Thorn, N. A. (1965). The effects of calcium on protein-binding and metabolism of arginine–vasopressin in rats. *J. Endocr.* **32,** 141–151.

Solomon, A. K. (1960). Pores in the cell membrane. *Scient. Am.* **203,** 146–150.

Solomon, S. (1957). Transtubular potential differences of rat kidney. *J. cell. comp. Physiol.* **49,** 351–357.

Sperber, I. (1944). Studies on the mammalian kidney. *Zool. Bidr. Upps.* **22,** 249–431.

Stadie, W. O. & Riggs, B. C. (1944). Microtome for the preparation of tissue slices for metabolic studies of surviving tissues *in vitro*. *J. biol. Chem.* **154,** 687–690.

Stannier, M. W. (1960). The function of the mammalian mesonephros. *J. Physiol.* **151,** 472–478.

— (1969). Micropuncture of nephrons of new-born pig. *J. Physiol.* **200,** 24P.

Starling, E. H. (1899). The glomerular function of the kidney. *J. Physiol.* **24,** 317–330.

Starling, E. H. & Verney, E. B. (1925). The secretion of urine as studied on the isolated kidney. *Proc. Roy. Soc.* **B97,** 321–363.

Stephenson, J. L. (1965). Ability of counterflow systems to concentrate. *Nature, Lond.* **206,** 1215–1219.

— (1966). Concentration in renal counterflow systems. *Biophys. J.* **6,** 539–542.

Sutherland, E. W. & Rall, T. W. (1960). The relation of adenosine 3′,5′-phosphate and phosphorylase to the actions of catecholamines and other hormones. *Pharmac. Rev.* **12,** 265–299.

Swan, A. G. & Miller, A. T. (1960). Osmotic regulation in isolated liver and kidney slices. *Am. J. Physiol.* **199,** 1227–1231.

Takahashi, K., Kamimura, M., Shinko, T. & Tsuji, S. (1966). Effects of vasopressin and water load on urinary adenosine 3′,5′ cyclic mono-phosphate. *Lancet* **ii,** 967–969.

Tata, P., Heller, J. & Gauer, O. H. (1965). Uber die antidiuretische Aktivität in der Lymphe von Katzen. *Pflüger's Arch. ges. Physiol.* **283,** 222–229.

Thoburn, G. D., Kopald, H. H., Herd, J. A., Hollenberg, M., O'Morchoe, C. C. & Barger, A. C. (1963). Intrarenal distribution of nutrient blood flow determined with [85]Kr in the unanaesthetized dog. *Circulation Res.* **13,** 290–312.

Thorn, N. A. (1960). An effect of antidiuretic hormone on renal excretion of calcium in dogs. *Dan. med. Bull.* **7,** 110–113.

Thorn, N. A., Knudsen, P. J. & Koefoed, J. (1961). Antidiuretic effect of large doses of bovine testicular hyaluronidase in rats. *Acta endocr.* **38,** 571–576.

Thorn, N. A. & Silver, L. (1957). Chemical form of circulating anti-diuretic hormone in rats. *J. exp. Med.* **105**, 575–583.

Thorn, N. A. & Smith, M. W. (1965). Renal excretion of synthetic arginine–vasopressin injected into dogs. *Acta endocr.* **49**, 388–392.

Thurau, K. (1966). Influence of sodium concentration at macula densa cells on tubular sodium load. *Ann. N.Y. Acad. Sci.* **139**, 388–399.

Thurau, K., Deetjen, P. & Güntzler, H. (1962). Die diurese bei arteriellen Drucksteigerungen. *Pflüger's Arch. ges. Physiol.* **274**, 567–580.

Thurau, K., Deetjen, P. & Kramer, K. (1960). Hämodynamik des Nierenmarks. *Pflüger's Arch. ges. Physiol.* **270**, 270–285.

Thurau, K. & Schnermann, J. (1965). Die Natriumkonzentration an den Macula densa Zellen als regulierender Faktor für das Glomerulumfiltrat (Mikropunktionsversuche). *Klin. Wschr.* **43**, 110.

Thurau, K., Wilde, W. S., Henne, G., Schnermann, J. & Prčhal, K. (1963). Flow dynamics in the inner part of the medulla: protein concentration in vasa recta and urine flow rates in the loops of Henle. *Proc. 2nd int. Congr. Nephrology, Pague.*

Torelli, G., Milla, E., Faelli, A. & Constantini, S. (1966). Energy requirement for sodium reabsorption in the *in vivo* rabbit kidney. *Am. J. Physiol.* **211**, 576–580.

Towbin, E. J. & Ferrell, C. B. (1963). Stop flow study of renal excretion of tritiated vasopressin. *J. clin. Invest.* **42**, 987–992.

Trueta, J., Barclay, A. E., Daniel, P. M., Franklin, K. J. & Prichard, M. M. L. (1947). *Studies of the Renal Circulation.* Oxford: Blackwell.

Ullrich, K. J. (1959). Das Nierenmark. Struktur, Stoffwechsel und Funktion. *Ergebn. Physiol.* **50**, 433–489.

— (1962). Direct evidence for a sodium chloride pumping mechanism in the thin Henle's loop and for a relatively small *in vivo* glycolysis in the kidney medulla. *Proc. XXII int. Congr. Physiol., Leiden,* vol. I, pp. 367–369. Intern. Congress Series. Amsterdam.

Ullrich, K. J., Drenckhahn, F. R. & Jarausch, K. H. (1955). Untersuchungen zum Problem der Harnkonzentrierung und verdunnung: über des osmotische Verhalten von Nierenzellen und die begleitende Elektrolytanhaufung im Nierengewebe bei verschiedenen Diuresezustanden. *Pflüger's Arch. ges. Physiol.* **261**, 62–77.

Ullrich, K. J. & Eigler, F. W. (1958). Sekretion von Wasserstoffionen in dem Samelröhren der Saügetierniere. *Pflüger's Arch. ges. Physiol.* **267**, 491–496.

Ullrich, K. J., Jarausch, K. H. (1956). Uber Verteilung von Elektrolyten (Na, K, Ca, Mg, Cl, anorganischem Phosphat) Harnstoff, Aminosäuren, exogenen Kreatinin und organischen Phosphorverbindungen in Rinde und Mark der Hundeniere bei verschiedenen Diuresezustanden. *Proc. XXe Congr. int. Physiol., Bruxelles.* pp. 92–93.

Ullrich, K. J., Jarausch, K. H. & Overbeck, W. (1955). Verteiling von Na, K, Ca, Mg, Cl, PO$_4$ und Harnstoff in Rinde und Mark der Hundeniere bei verschiedenen Funktionzustanden *Ber. ges. Physiol. exp. Pharm.* **180**, 131–139.

Ullrich, K. J. & Marsh, D. J. (1963). Kidney, water and electrolyte metabolism. *Ann. Rev. Physiol.* **25**, 91–142.

Ullrich, K. J., Pehling, G. & Espinar-Lafuente, M. (1961). Wasser- und der Elektrolytfluss im vaskularen Gegenströmsystem des Nierenmarks. *Pflüger's Arch. ges. Physiol.* **273**, 562–572.

Ullrich, K. J., Pehling, G. & Stockle, H. (1961). Hämoglobinkonzentration Erythrocytenzahl und Hämatocrit im vasa recta blut. *Pflügers Arch. ges. Physiol.* **273**, 573–578.

Ullrich, K. J. & Rumrich, G. (1963). Direkte Messung der Wasserpermeabilität corticaler Nephronabschnitte bei verschiedenen Diuresezustanden. *Pflüger's Arch. ges. Physiol.* **278**, 44R.

Ullrich, K. J., Rumrich, G. & Fuchs, G. (1966). Wasserpermeabilität und transtubularer Wasserfluss corticaler Nephronsabschnitte bei verschiedenen Diuresezustanden. *Pflügers Arch. ges. Physiol.* **280**, 99–119.

Ullrich, K. J., Schmidt-Nielsen, B., O'Dell, R., Pehling, G., Gottschalk, C. W., Lassiter, W. E. & Mylle, M. (1963). Micropuncture study of composition of proximal and distal tubular fluid in rat kidney. *Am. J. Physiol.* **204**, 527–531.

Van Dyke, H. B., Chow, B. F., Greep, R. O. & Rothen, A. (1942). The isolation of a protein from the pars neuralis of the ox pituitary with constant oxytocic, pressor and diuresis-inhibiting activities. *J. Pharmac.* **74**, 190–209.

Vurek, G. G. & Bowman, R. L. (1965). Helium-glow photometer for picomole analysis of alkali metals. *Science, N.Y.* **149**, 448–450.

Wachstein, M. & Bradshaw, M. (1965). Histochemical localization of enzyme activity in the kidneys of three mammalian species during their postnatal development. *J. Histochem. Cytochem.* **13**, 44–56.

Walker, A. M. (1930). Comparisons of total molecular concentration of glomerular urine and blood plasma from the frog and from *Necturus*. *J. biol. Chem.* **87**, 499–522.

— (1933). Quantitative studies of the composition of glomerular urine —X. The concentration of inorganic phosphate in glomerular urine from frogs and *Necturi* determined by an ultramicromodification of the Bell–Doisy method. *J. biol. Chem.* **101**, 239–254.

Walker, A. M., Bott, P. A., Oliver, J. & McDowell, M. C. (1941). The collection and analysis of fluid from single nephrons of the mammalian kidney. *Am. J. Physiol.* **134**, 580–595.

Walker, A. M. & Elsom, K. A. (1930). A quantitative study of the glomerular elimination of urea in frogs. *J. biol. Chem.* **91**, 593–616.

Walker, A. M. & Hudson, C. L. (1937a). The reabsorption of glucose from the renal tubule in amphibia and the action of phlorizin upon it. *Am. J. Physiol.* **118**, 130–143.

— (1937b). The role of the tubule in the excretion of urea by the amphibian kidney. *Am. J. Physiol.* **118**, 167–173.

Walker, A. M. & Oliver, J. (1941). Methods for the collection of fluid from single glomeruli and tubules of the mammalian kidney. *Am. J. Physiol.* **134**, 562–571.

Walker, A. M. & Reisinger, J. A. (1933). Quantitative studies of the composition of glomerular urine—IX. The concentration of reducing substances in glomerular urine from frogs and *Necturi* determined by an ultramicroadaptation of the method of Sumner. Observations on the action of phlorizin. *J. biol. Chem.* **101**, 223–238.

Walter, R., Rudinger, J. & Schwartz, I. L. (1967). Chemistry and structure-activity relations of the antidiuretic hormones. *Am. J. Med.* **42**, 653–677.

Wearn, J. T. & Richards, A. N. (1924). Observations on the composition of glomerular urine, with particular reference to the problem of reabsorption in the renal tubules. *Am. J. Physiol.* **71**, 209–227.

— (1925). The concentration of chlorides in the glomerular urine of frogs. *J. biol. Chem.* **66**, 247–273.

Weaver, A. N., McCarver, C. T. & Swann, H. G. (1956). Distribution of blood in the functional kidney. *J. exp. Med.* **104**, 41–52.

Weinstein, S. W. & Klose, R. M. (1969). Micropuncture studies on energy metabolism and sodium transport in the mammalian nephron. *Am. J. Physiol.* **217**, 498–504.

Wesson, L. G. & Anslow, W. P. (1948). Excretion of sodium and water during osmotic diuresis in the dog. *Am. J. Physiol.* **153**, 465–474.

— (1952). Effect of osmotic and mercurial diuresis on simultaneous water diuresis. *Am. J. Physiol.* **170**, 255–269.

Wesson, L. G., Anslow, W. P. & Smith, H. W. (1948). The excretion of strong electrolytes. *Bull. N.Y. Acad. Med.* **24**, 586–606.

West, C. D., Kaplan, S. A., Fomon, S. J. & Rapoport, S. (1952). Urine flow and solute excretion during osmotic diuresis in hydrated dogs: role of distal tubule in the production of hypotonic urine. *Am. J. Physiol.* **170**, 239–254.

Westfall, B. B., Findley, T. & Richards, A. N. (1934). Quantitative studies of the composition of glomerular urine—XII. The concentration of chloride in glomerular urine of frogs and *Necturi*. *J. biol. Chem.* **107**, 661–672.

Whitlock, R. T. & Wheeler, H. O. (1964). Coupled transport of solute and water across rabbit gallbladder epithelium. *J. clin. Invest.* **43**, 2249–2265.

Whittembury, G. & Windhager, E. E. (1961). Electrical potential difference measurements in perfused single proximal tubules of *Necturus* kidney. *J. gen. Physiol.* **44**, 679–687.

Widdowson, E. M. & Spray, C. M. (1951). Chemical development in utero. *Arch. Dis. Childh.* **26**, 205–214.

Wiederholt, M., Hierholzer, K., Windhager, E. E. & Giebisch, G. (1957). Microperfusion study of fluid reabsorption in proximal tubules of rat kidneys. *Am. J. Physiol.* **213**, 809–818.

Wilde, W. S. & Vorburger, C. (1967). Albumen multiplier in kidney vasa recta analysed by microspectrophotometry of T–1824. *Amer. J. Physiol.* **213**, 1233–1243.

Windhager, E. E. (1965). Electrophysiological study of the renal papilla of Golden Hamsters. *Am. J. Physiol.* **206**, 694–700.

Windhager, E. E. & Giebisch, G. (1961). Micropuncture study of renal tubular transfer of sodium chloride in the rat. *Am. J. Physiol.* **200**, 581–590.

Windhager, E. E., Whittembury, G., Oken, D. E., Schatzmann, H. J. & Solomon, A. K. (1959). Single proximal tubules of the *Necturus* kidney. Dependence of H_2O movement on NaCl concentration. *Am. J. Physiol.* **197**, 313–325.

Windle, W. F. (1940). *The Physiology of the Foetus.* Philadelphia: Saunders.

Winton, F. R. (1931a). The influence of increase of ureter pressure on the isolated mammalian kidney. *J. Physiol.* **71**, 381–390.

— (1931b). The influence of venous pressure on the isolated mammalian kidney. *J. Physiol.* **72**, 49–61.

— (1931c). The glomerular pressure in the isolated mammalian kidney. *J. Physiol.* **72**, 361–375.

Wirz, H. (1953). Der osmotische Druck des Blutes in der Nieren-papille. *Helv. physiol. Pharmac. Acta* **11**, 20–29.

— (1956). Der osmotische Druk in den corticalen Tubuli der Rattenniere. *Helvet. physiol. Pharmac. Acta.* **14**, 353–362.

Wirz, H., Hargitay, B. & Kuhn, W. (1951). Lokalisation des Konzen-trierungsprozesses in der Niere durch direkte Kryoscopie. *Helv. physiol. Pharmac. Acta.* **9**, 195–207.

Wright, F. S., Knox, F. G., Howards, S. S. & Berliner, R. W. (1969). Reduced sodium reabsorption by the proximal tubule of DOCA-escaped dogs. *Am. J. Physiol.* **216**, 869–875.

Zadunaisky, J. A. & De Fisch, F. W. (1964). Active and passive chloride movements across isolated amphibian skin. *Am. J. Physiol.* **207**, 1010–1014.

Zak, G. A., Brun, C. & Smith, H. W. (1954). The mechanism of formation of osmotically concentrated urine during antidiuretic state. *J. clin. Invest.* **33**, 1064–1074.

AUTHOR INDEX

HÜMMEL, R.   *29, 30*

ISAACSON, L.   Burg, M. B., ——, Grantham, J. & Orloff, J. *47*
ISHIDA, Y.   & Hara, K. *115*
IVANOVA, L. N.   Ginetzinsky, A. G. & —— *109*
IVANOVA, L. N.   Ginetzinsky, A. G., Broytman, A. E. & —— *109*
IVERSON, D. A.   Nungesser, W. C., Pfeiffer, E. W., —— & Wallerius, J. F. *25*
IVERSON, D. A.   Pfeiffer, E. W., Nungesser, W. C., —— & Wallerius, J. F. *17, 21, 22, 27, 28, 30*

JAMISON, R. L.   Bennett, C. M. & Berliner, R. W. *87, 89, 90, 91, 92, 93, 94, 95, 96, 156*
JAMISON, R. L.   Sakai, F., —— & Berliner, R. W. *87*
JARAUSCH, K. H.   & Ullrich, K. J. *42*
JARAUSCH, K. H.   Ullrich, K. J. & —— *37*
JARAUSCH, K. H.   Ullrich, K. J., —— & Overbeck, W. *37*
JARAUSCH, K. H.   Ullrich, K. J., Drenckhahn, F. O. & —— *25, 36, 37, 42, 151*
JARD, S.   & Morel, F. *114, 115, 116, 121*
JAYASENA, K.   Ginsburg, M. & —— *145*
JONES, A. M.   & Schlapp, W. *112*
JONES, C. B.   Baer, J. E., ——, Spitzer, A. S. & Russo, H. F. *102*
JONES, J. J.   Harvey, N., —— & Lee, J. *112, 113*
JOŠT, K.   Rudinger, J. & —— *115, 122*

KAIM, J. T.   Brodsky, W. A., Miley, J. F., —— & Shah, N. P. *86*
KAMIMURA, M.   Takahashi, K., ——, Shinko, T. & Tsuji, S. *129*
KAPLAN, A.   Freidman, M. & Kruger, H. E. *24*
KAPLAN, S. A.   West, C. D., ——, Fomon, S. J. & Rapoport, S. *5*
KASHGARIAN, M.   Stoeckle, H., Gottschalk, C. W. & Ullrich, K. J. *47, 49*
KASHGARIAN, M.   Hayslett, J. P., —— & Epstein, F. H. *56*
KATCHALSKY, A.   Kedem, O. & —— *99*
KAUFMAN, J. J.   Goodwin, H. E. & —— *24*
KAYE, G. I.   Wheeler, H. O., Whitlock, R. T. & Lane, N. *109*
KEDEM, O.   & Katchalsky, A. *99*
KEDEM, O.   Civan, M. M., —— & Leaf, A. *100*
KELLER, W.   György, P., —— & Brehme, T. *87*
KELLOG, R. H.   Koike, T. I. & —— *87*
KELMAN, R. B.   *49, 50*
KERR, W. S.   Leaf, A., ——, Wrong, O. & Chatillon, J. Y. *10*
KERRIDGE, P. M. T.   Bayliss, L. E., —— & Russell, D. S. *2*
KEYL, M. J.   Henry, L. P., —— & Bell, R. D. *26*
KING, V. M.   Dicker, S. E. & —— *145*
KITTELSON, J. A.   *16, 134*
KLEEMAN, C. R.   Czaczkes, J. W. & —— *112*
KLEEMAN, C. R.   Cutler, R. E., ——, Maxwell, M. H. & Dowling, J. T. *117*
KLEIN, E.   Burdon-Sandersen, J., Foster, M. & Brunton, T. L. *136*
KLOSE, R. M.   Giebisch, G., —— & Windhager, E. E., *49, 54*

SMITH, H. W.	*4, 5, 6, 8, 9, 10, 11, 15, 16, 17, 27, 32, 58, 73, 80, 96, 97, 149*
SMITH, H. W.	Marshall, E. K. & —— *17*
SMITH, H. W.	Wesson, L. G., Anslow, W. P. & —— *7*
SMITH, H. W.	Zak, G. A., Brun, C. & —— *11*
SMITH, M. W.	& Sachs, H. *115*
SMITH, M. W.	& Thorn, N. A. *112, 113*
SMITH, M. W.	Thorn, N. A. & —— *112*
SMITH-AGREDA, V.	Diepen, R., Engelhardt, F. & —— *145*
SNAITH, A. H.	Orr, J. & —— *112*
SOLOMON, A. K.	*47*
SOLOMON, A. K.	Maude, D. L., Shehadeh, J. & —— *46*
SOLOMON, A. K.	Windhager, E. E., Whittemburg, G., Oken, D E., Schatzmann, H. J. & —— *45*
SOLOMON, S.	*98*
SOLOMON, S.	Marsh, D. J. & —— *82*
SPERBER, I.	*17, 22, 27, 30, 152*
SPITZER, A. S.	Baer, J. E., Jones, C. B., —— & Russo, H. F. *102*
SPRAY, C. M.	Widdowson, E. M. & —— *136*
STADIE, W. O.	& Riggs, B. C. *145*
STANIER, M. W.	*133, 148*
STANIER, M. W.	McCance, R. A. & —— *133, 137*
STARLING, E. H.	*2*
STARLING, E. H.	& Verney, E. B. *2*
STEPHENSON, J. L.	*74, 75, 156*
STÖCKLE, H.	Ullrich, K. J., Pehling, G. & —— *23*
STOECKLE, H.	Kashgarian, M., ——, Gottschalk, C. W. & Ullrich, K. J. *47, 49*
STOUFFER, J. E.	Aroskar, J. P., Chan, W. Y., ——, Schneider, C. H., Murti, V. V. S. & Du Vigneaud, V. *112*
SULLIVAN, R.	Bergen, S. S., ——, Hilton, J. G., Willis, S. W. & Van Itallie, T. B. *128*
SULLIVAN, L. P.	Malvin, R. L., Wilde, W. S., & —— *7*
SUTHERLAND, E. W.	& Rall, T. W. *128*
SUTHERLAND, E. W.	Butcher, R. W. & —— *129*
SUTHERLAND, E. W.	Handler, J. S., Butcher, R. W., —— & Orloff, J. *129*
SWAN, A. G	& Miller, A. T. *33*
SWANN, H. G.	Nanninga, L. B., —— & Schubert, M. L. *23*
SWANN, H. G.	Weaver, A. N., McCarver, C. T. & —— *22*
TATA, P.	Heller, J. & Gauer, O. H. *113*
TAKAHASHI, K.	Kamimura, M., Shinko, R. & Tsuji, S. *129*
THOBURN, G. D.	Kopald, H. H., Herd, J. A., Hollenberg, M, O'Morchoe, C. C. & Barger, A. C. *24*
THOBURN, G. D.	Herd, J. A., Hollenberg, M., ——, Kopald, H. H. & Barger, A. C. *23*
THORN, N. A.	*110*
THORN, N. A.	Knudsen, P. J. & Koefoed, J. *110*
THORN, N. A.	& Silver, L. *113*
THORN, N. A.	& Smith, M. W. *112*
THORN, N. A.	Smith, M. W. & —— *112, 113*
THURAU, K.	*50, 51*

WILDE, W. S.   & Vorburger, C. *157*
WILKINSON, E.   McCance, R. A. & —— *137*
WILLIS, S. W.   Bergen, S. S., Sullivan, R., Hilton, J. G., —— &
                       Van Itallie, T. B., *128*
WINDHAGER, E. E.   *83*
WINDHAGER, E. E.   & Giebisch, G. *47, 53*
WINDHAGER, E. E.   Giebisch, G. & —— *47, 48, 49, 57*
WINDHAGER, E. E.   Giebisch, G., Klose, R. M. & —— *49, 54*
WINDHAGER, E. E.   Wiederholt, M., Hierholzer, K., —— & Giebisch,
                       G. *52*
WINDHAGER, E. E.   Whittembury, G. & —— *47*
WINDHAGER, E. E.   Whittembury, G., Oken, D. E., Schatzmann,
                       H. J. & Solomon, A. K. *45*
WINDLE, W. F.   *133*
WINGATE, D. L.   Parsons, D. S. & —— *13*
WINTERS, R. W.   Scaglione, P. R., Dell, R. B. & —— *93*
WINTON, F. R.   *2*
WIRZ, H.   *9, 39, 41, 42, 47, 53, 97, 105*
WIRZ, H.   Hargitay, B. & Kuhn, W. *33, 36, 73*
WIRZ, H.   Hargitay, B., Kuhn, W. & —— *67, 69, 73*
WRIGHT, F. S.   Knox, F. G., Howards, S. S. & Berliner, R. W. *53*
WRONG, O.   Leaf, A., Kerr, W. S., —— & Chatillon, J. Y. *10*

YALLOW, A. A.   Goldman, A. G., —— & Grossman, J. *57*
YELINEK, L.   Ruiz-Guinazu, A., Arrizurieta, E. E. & —— *37*
YOFFEY, J. M.   Baxter, J. S. & —— *134*
YOUNG, R.   Rasmussen, H., Schwartz, I. L., —— & Marc-
                       Aurele, J. *117*

ZADUNAISKY, J. A.   & De Fisch, F. W. *49*
ZAIDI, S. M.   Heller, H. & —— *117*
ZAIMIS, E. J.   Heller, H. & —— *142*
ZAK, G. A.   Brun, C. & Smith, H. W. *11*
ZAK, G. A.   Page, L. B., Scott-Baker, J. C., ——, Becker,
                       E. L. & Baxter, C. F. *11*

SUBJECT INDEX

'Single effect', countercurrent system and, **65**
thin ascending limb reabsorption of Na as, 90–91
Sodium, concentration in loop of Henle and collecting duct of, 40
  concentration in papillary tissue and in urine of, 37
  G.F.R. control by concentration at macula densa of, 50–51
  loop of Henle reabsorption of, 53–54
  medullary gradient of osmolarity and, **42**
  proximal tubule reabsorption of, 45–**48**
Sodium excretion, mannitol diuresis effect on, 12
Sodium pump, ADH action on, 99–100
Sodium transport, vasopressin possible action on, 156
Solvent drag, membrane permeability and, 104
Species difference, in ADH action on distal tubule, 105
  in length of loop of Henle, 17
  in medulla/cortex thickness ratio, **25**
  in nephron numbers, 16
  in osmotic gradient of kidney slices, 38–**39**
  in presence of papilla and shape of renal pelvis, 27–28
  in proportion of injected vasopressin excreted, 112
  in renal function in new-born, 134–136
  in U/P maximum osmolar concentration, 11
  in vasa recta distribution, 20–**21**
'Stopped flow microperfusion', proximal tubule reabsorption of Na investigated by, 45–46
Sulphydryl reagents, vasopressin action on amphibian bladder inhibition by, 118

Theophylline, vasopressin-like activity of, 128
Toad, vasopressin effect on water uptake from various solutions by, **126**
Toad bladder, ADH action on, 99
  sodium transport by, 102–103
Toad skin, barriers of water and solute entry through, 100
Tritiated water, equilibration time of cortex and medulla for injected, 84
Tropical bovids, medulla/cortex thickness ratio and maximum concentration in, 29
Tubules, development in new-born of, 135

U/P osmolarity ratio, species difference in maximum, 11
Urea, ADH action on permeability of collecting duct to, **107**
  concentration in different regions of nephron of, 58–59
  concentration in loop of Henle and collecting duct of, 40
  gradient in medulla of, 37
  toad bladder permeation by, 99
Urine concentration, classical theory of mechanism of, 15
Urine flow, G.F.R. in new-born and adult relation to, **147**
  osmolar concentration relation to, **2**
Urine osmolarity, medulla/cortex thickness ratio relation to maximum, **25–26**

Vasa recta, countercurrent exchange system role of, 95
  osmolar concentration in ascending and descending limbs and in, 89
  osmolar concentration of urine and blood from loop of, 39–40
  pressure fall in, **84**